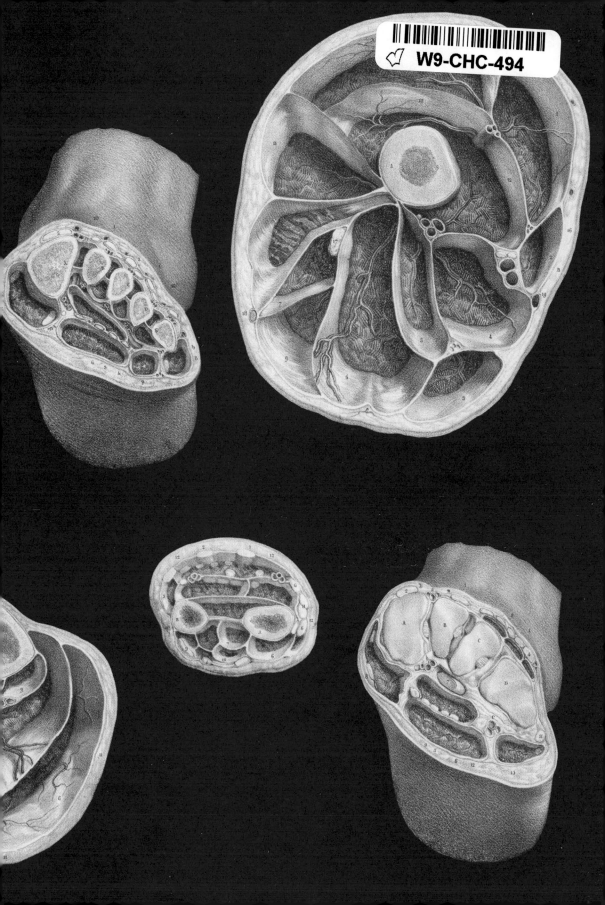

W9-CHC-494

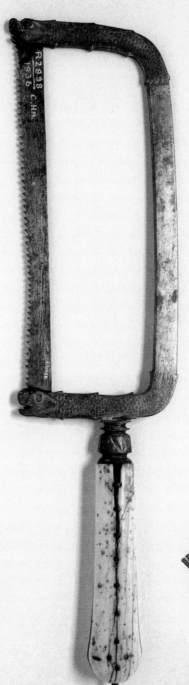

WITHDRAWN FROM LIBRARY

Pl. 2.

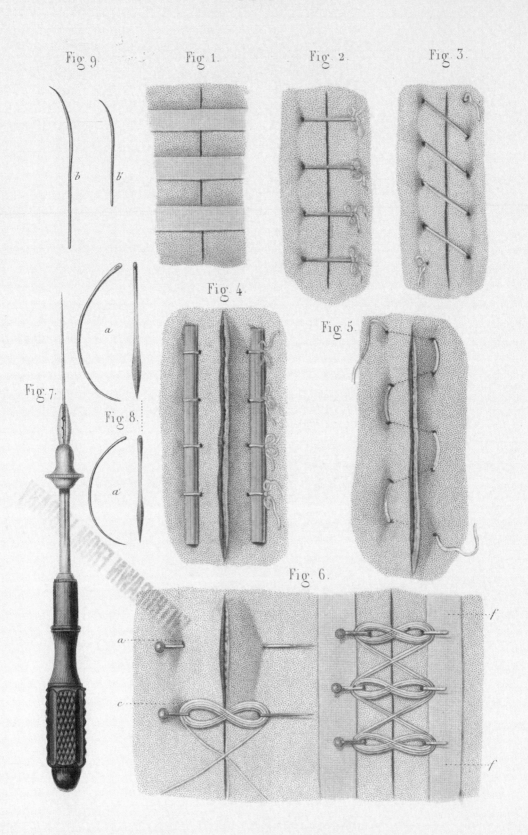

Fig. 9.   Fig. 1.   Fig. 2.   Fig. 3.

Fig. 4.

Fig. 5.

Fig. 7.

Fig. 8.

Fig. 6.

MONTGOMERY COLLEGE
ROCKVILLE CAMPUS LIBRARY
ROCKVILLE, MARYLAND

CRUCIAL

INTERVENTIONS

AN

ILLUSTRATED TREATISE

ON THE

PRINCIPLES & PRACTICE

OF

NINETEENTH-CENTURY

SURGERY.

BY RICHARD BARNETT

WITH A FOREWORD BY

PROFESSOR ROGER L. KNEEBONE

PHD FRCS FRCSED FRCGP

THAMES & HUDSON LTD.

M M X V

3562052

APR 11 2017

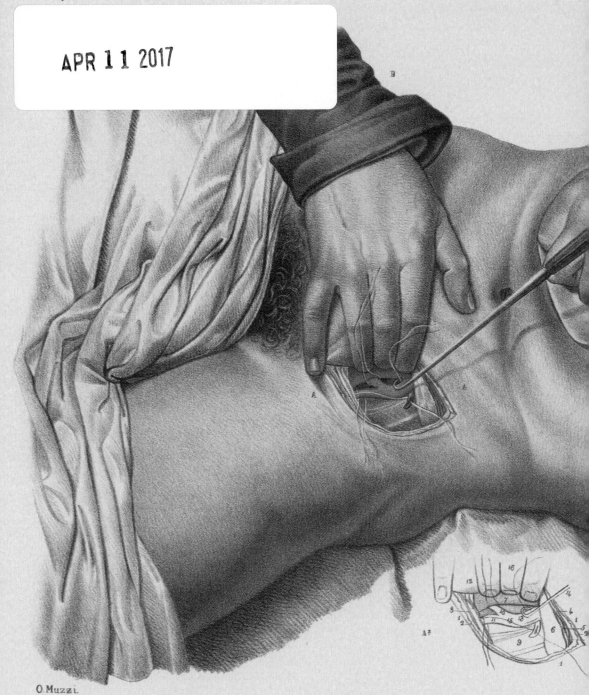

O.Muzzi.

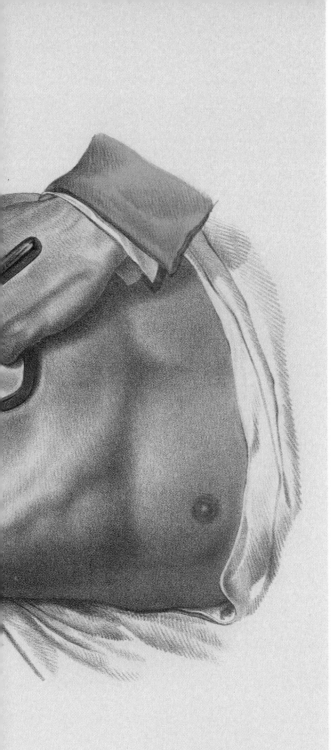

Li t Rdolfi.

FRONT COVER: A method of stemming bleeding from the carotid and axillary arteries of the head and neck, using straps, pads, and a compression clamp to apply pressure. BACK COVER: Various techniques for amputation of the hand, foot, fingers and toes. (*page 1*) A small bow-framed amputation saw, *c.* 1580, ivory-handled, with an ornate design on its damascened frame. (*page 2*) Various techniques for suturing skin wounds, with a selection of needles and a needle-holder. (*This page*) Ligature of an artery in the inguinal region, using sutures and a suture hook, with compression of the abdomen to reduce aortic blood flow. (*pages 6–7*) Various surgical incisions produced by holding a scalpel in different positions. (*pages 8–9*) Various procedures for tenotomy (the cutting of a tendon to lengthen a muscle), along with illustrations of the underlying musculo-skeletal anatomy. (*page 11*) Dissection of the trunk of a man, showing the superficial organs of the thorax and abdomen. (*page 13*) Amputation of the leg at the tibiofemoral (knee) joint. (*page 14*) The title page of Johann Vesling's *Syntagma Anatomicum*, published 1647. Two female figures symbolize theoretical and practical anatomy; beyond them, Vesling conducts a dissection in the anatomy theatre at the University of Padua.

Crucial Interventions © 2015
Thames & Hudson Ltd, London

Design by Daniel Streat at Barnbrook

This book is published in partnership with Wellcome Collection and Wellcome Library, part of Wellcome Trust, 215 Euston Road, London NW1 2BE. www.wellcomecollection.org

wellcome collection

Wellcome Collection is part of Wellcome Trust, a global charitable foundation dedicated to achieving extraordinary improvements in human and animal health. Wellcome Trust is a charity registered in England and Wales, no. 210183.

All the images reproduced in this book are reproduced courtesy of the Wellcome Library, except where stated. For further information about individual images, see pages 250–53.

All Rights Reserved. No part of this publication may be reproduced or transmitted in any form or by any means, electronic or mechanical, including photocopy, recording or any other information storage and retrieval system, without prior permission in writing from the publisher.

First published in 2015 in hardcover in the United States of America by Thames & Hudson Inc., 500 Fifth Avenue, New York, New York 10110

thamesandhudsonusa.com

Library of Congress Catalog Card Number 2015932470

ISBN 978-0-500-51810-6

Printed and bound in China by Everbest Printing Co. Ltd

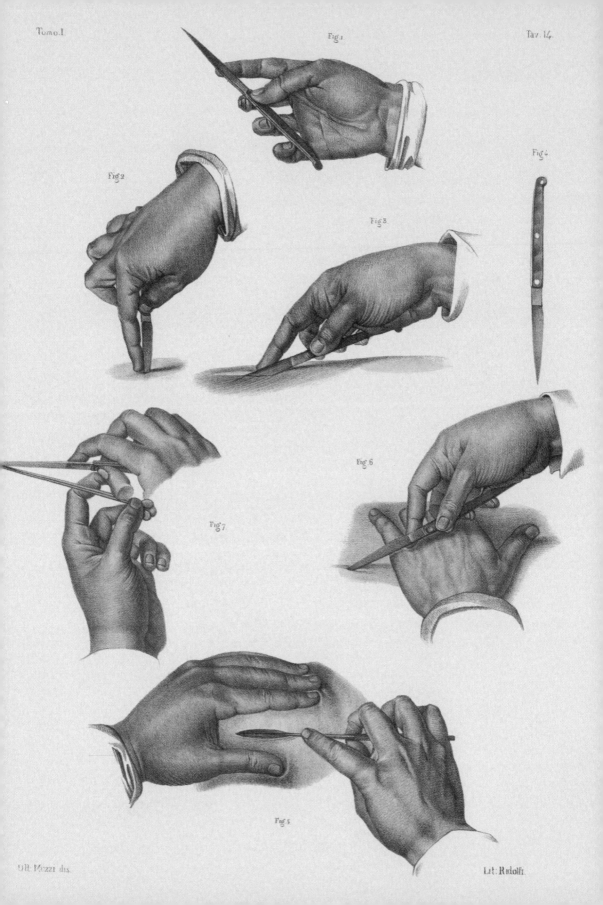

Fig.1

Fig.4

Fig.2

Fig.3

Fig.6

Fig.7

Fig.5

OR. Mezzi dis.

Lit: Rudolfi.

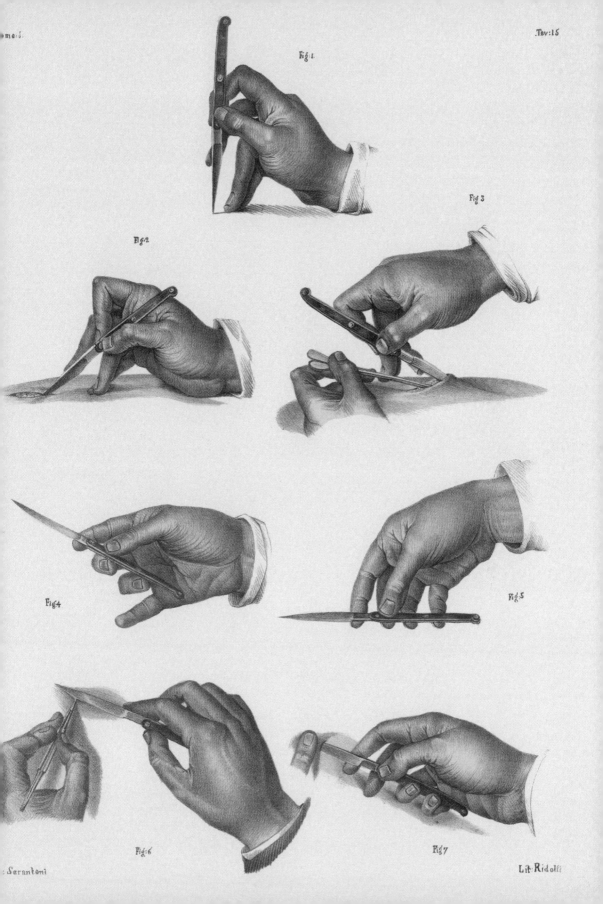

Fig:1.

Fig 3

Fig:2

Fig4

Fig:5

Fig:6

Fig:7

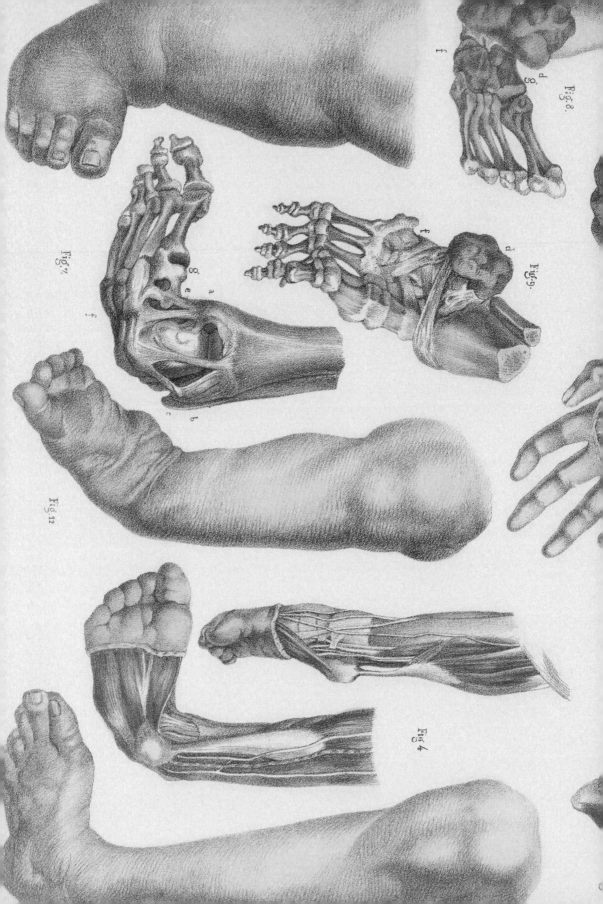

Fig.8.

Fig.9.

Fig.7.

Fig 12

Fig 4

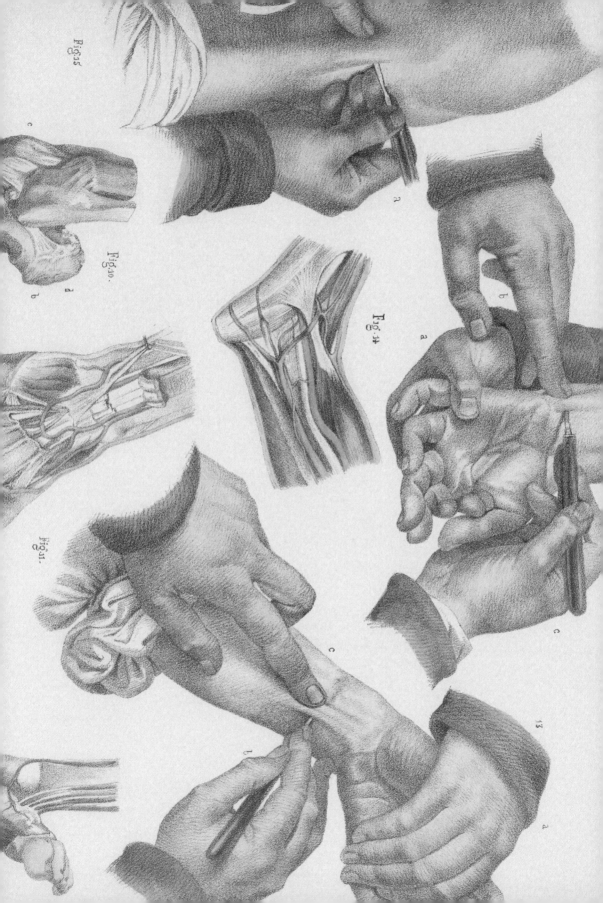

Fig.35.

Fig.30.

Fig.34.

Fig.31.

13

CONTENTS.

FOREWORD by Professor Roger L. Kneebone 12

INTRODUCTION The Thinking Hand:
Surgery as Craft, Art & Science 14

Head & Neck

I.   HEAD 46

II.   EYES 70

III. EAR, NOSE & THROAT 96

Upper Body

IV.   HANDS & ARMS 122

V.   CHEST 148

VI.   ABDOMEN 166

Lower Body

VII. GENITALS 188

VIII. LEGS & FEET 216

Further Reading 246
Picture Credits 250
Index 254
About the Author / Acknowledgments 256

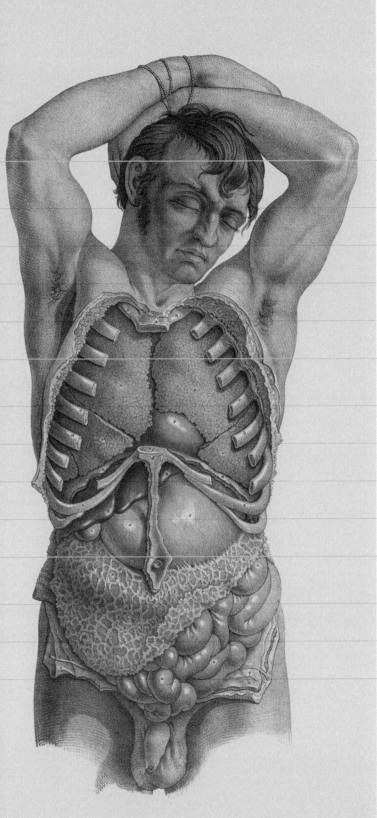

ARTICLES.

A. *The Yankee Dodge:*   64
Anaesthesia.

B. *Let us Spray:*   90
Antisepsis & the Hospital.

C. *Scrubbing Up:*   116
Asepsis & the Operating Theatre.

D. *Ministers of Hygiene:*   142
Surgery & Nursing.

E. *The Smart of the Knife:*   160
Surgery & War.

F. *Walking the Wards:*   182
Teaching & Organizing Surgery.

G. *So Simple & So Grand:*   210
Surgery in 1900.

H. *Under the Knife:*   240
The Patient's Perspective.

I N *CRUCIAL INTERVENTIONS*, RICHARD BARNETT TURNS WITH CHARACTERISTIC LUCIDITY TO THE WORLD OF NINETEENTH-CENTURY SURGERY, EXPOSING ITS TENSIONS AND CONTRADICTIONS WITH MERCILESS PRECISION. A COMPELLING FUSION OF NARRATIVE AND ILLUSTRATION INVITES US TO LOOK WITH FRESH EYES AT THIS MOST FASCINATING OF CENTURIES.

THE BOOK HAS PROMPTED ME TO THINK BACK OVER MY OWN CAREER IN SURGERY. DURING THE MANY YEARS I SPENT MASTERING THE 'MECHANICAL ART' OF MY PROFESSION, THE OPERATING THEATRE SEEMED A PLACE OF STABILITY. THINGS, IT SEEMED TO ME THEN, MUST ALWAYS HAVE BEEN AS I EXPERIENCED THEM AS AN INSIDER. IT TAKES A HISTORIAN'S DETACHMENT TO POINT OUT THE RICH AND CONTESTED BACKSTORIES THAT SEETHE UNDERNEATH THE COOL, CLINICAL TERRITORIES OF SURGERY. *CRUCIAL INTERVENTIONS* TELLS THOSE STORIES.

THE BOOK'S INTRODUCTION, ENTITLED *THE THINKING HAND: SURGERY AS CRAFT, ART & SCIENCE*, SETS OUT BARNETT'S SCOPE. IN A SKILFUL SYNTHESIS OF MEDICAL AND HISTORICAL PERSPECTIVES, HE DISCLOSES POWERFUL AND CONFLICTING CURRENTS WITHIN SURGICAL PRACTICE ACROSS EUROPE. IN THE EIGHT SHORT ESSAYS THAT FOLLOW, BARNETT PRESENTS A CAREFULLY CHOSEN SERIES OF PROVOCATIONS THAT GUIDE THE READER THROUGH THE COMPLEX ISSUES OF THE TIME, AND UNWRAPS THEM UNDER A VERY TWENTY-FIRST-CENTURY LENS.

LIKE ITS PREDECESSOR, *THE SICK ROSE*, THIS BOOK COMBINES A GRIPPING NARRATIVE WITH BEAUTIFUL AND OFTEN UNCOMFORTABLE ILLUSTRATIONS DRAWN FROM WELLCOME'S UNIQUE COLLECTIONS. THOUGH ALWAYS ERUDITE, BARNETT WEARS HIS SCHOLARSHIP LIGHTLY, AND HIS ARGUMENTS ARE BOTH ELOQUENT AND PERSUASIVE. THIS IS A BOOK TO BE SAVOURED.

PROFESSOR ROGER L. KNEEBONE
PHD FRCS FRCSED FRCGP

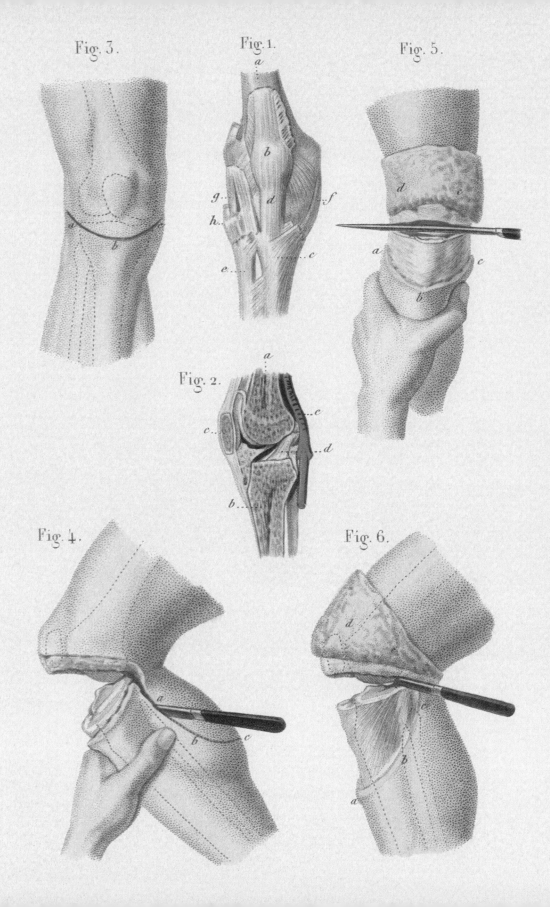

Fig. 3.

Fig. 1.

Fig. 5.

Fig. 2.

Fig. 4.

Fig. 6.

IOANNIS VESLINGII
MINDANI

SYNTAGMA
ANATOMICUM

PATAVII, cIɔIɔCXXXXVII
Typis Pauli Frambotti Bibliopolæ Sup. permissu.

Jo. Georgius Sculp.

THE THINKING HAND.

Surgery as Craft, Art & Science

L ooking back over a long and illustrious life, the Renaissance surgeon and anatomist Hieronymus Fabricius (also known as Girolamo Fabrizio) recalled one particularly notable operation. Some time in the late sixteenth century, a forty-year-old man had come to him in great pain—possibly with an infected wound or a tumour, more likely a broken bone. About to take the risky step of amputating his leg, Fabricius assembled his 'saw and Cauteries' and gathered a group of burly assistants to hold the man down while he worked. But things did not go quite as the surgeon had intended:

> *The sick man no sooner began to roare out, but all ranne away, except only my eldest Sonne, who was then but little, and to whom I had committed the holding of his thigh, for forme only; and but that my wife then great with child, came running out of the next chamber, and clapt hold of the Patient's Thorax, both he and myself had been in extreme danger.*

Fabricius' tale of heroism and agony captures so many of our assumptions about surgery in the age before anaesthesia and antisepsis. The blood and the bawling, the last-ditch butchery and the pervasive threat of death—all of this chimes beautifully with another classic representation of the surgeon in Johannes de Ketham's *Fasciculus Medicinae*, published c. 1493. In this illustration we see a medieval dissection: a physician, seated in a chair like a bishop's throne and clad in a sumptuous velvet robe and cap, reads from a text by Aristotle or Galen. Below him a surgeon, the sleeves of his doublet rolled up and a long, cruel knife in his hands, cuts open the corpse of an executed criminal. Ketham's woodcut is saturated with the symbolism of rank and status. The physician is above the surgeon in every sense: a scholar, a gentleman, heir to a long and learned tradition, his hands unsullied by the blood of the outcast dead. Here, in this one image, are all of the oppositions that run through histories of surgery: theory and practice, words and deeds, the head and the hand, the gentleman and the tradesman, the art of medicine and the craft of surgery. These oppositions have shaped our understanding of the nineteenth-century revolution in surgery—the subject of this book.

Well into the 1840s, Fabricius would have recognized much of what went on in those noisy, dirty, crowded spaces called operating theatres. Dressed in their street clothes, surgeons and assistants—all men—set to work on patients who remained awake throughout their ordeal. Operations were fast in the hope of minimizing pain, shock and blood loss, and mortality rates were high (though not so high as we might think). Yet within two generations operating theatres had come to resemble laboratories, with surgeons and female nurses clad in sterile gowns and working in near-silence. Anaesthesia had taken the problem of conscious patients out of the equation, and operations might take an hour or more; indeed, journalists were beginning to complain that new surgical

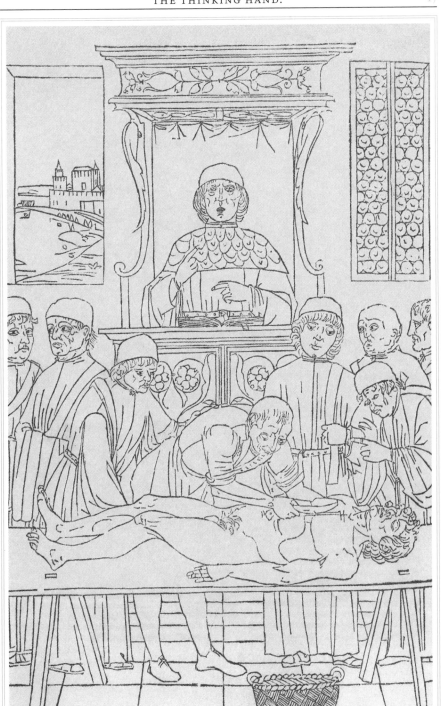

An early European anatomical dissection, from Johannes de Ketham's *Fasciculus Medicinae*, published *c.* 1493. A learned physician reads from a treatise while a surgeon carries out the dissection.

diagnoses, such as 'dropped kidneys', had been invented simply so that scalpel-happy surgeons could take a fee for operating. Surgeons entered culture and literature as High Victorian heroes and—in the formidable person of Joseph Lister, first Baron Lister of Lyme Regis—they also entered the aristocracy.

The roots of this revolution run deep, though, and their story takes us far beyond a simple set of oppositions between surgery and learned medicine. Fabricius himself shows us how complex early modern surgical identity could be. This crafty and quick-thinking surgeon also held a professorship at the University of Padua, one of the great centres of Renaissance medical thought. Contemporaries admired his skill and respected his erudition, and both he and his students—men such as William Harvey, the English physician who discovered the circulation of the blood—made major contributions to the 'New Anatomy' of the sixteenth and seventeenth centuries. Those who called themselves surgeons in Fabricius' time ranged from a handful of learned university professors, via guild and barber-surgeons working in towns, to a motley and diverse crew of oculists, bone-setters, monks in monastic infirmaries, and itinerants who specialized in the treatment of hernias, the reduction of dislocations, and the removal of bladder stones.

Turning this loose confederation of quarrelsome tribes into a single coherent Victorian profession called for a great deal of what sociologists call 'boundary-work'—drawing in those who sought respectability and unity, and keeping out those who might make trouble. To this end, surgery's past was reshaped to meet the demands of its present. Far from seeking to revive Classical practice—the great aim of their predecessors—eighteenth-century surgeons cast themselves in a heroic struggle to replace ignorance with hard-won empirical knowledge. This historical shift was charged with urgent contemporary purpose, as a justification for ambitious surgeons to move from the social and intellectual margins of medicine to its elite centre. It is a testament to their success that this remains the dominant public narrative of surgical history three centuries later.

The greatest challenge in telling the story of surgery lies in its very nature. Like ballet dancers or centre-forwards, surgeons rely on forms of expertise gained through experience and observation, which cannot easily be articulated. Does what surgeons know matter more than what they do? Has abstract learning driven refinements in operative technique, or have original ideas about the body emerged when surgeons tried new tricks, patients demanded new treatments, or when a culture's attitude to health and sickness began to change? The images collected here provide a magnificently rich resource with which to think about these questions and the visual, tactile, and sensual aspects of surgery, but the gap between what surgeons wrote—or, as we'll see, what others wrote about them—and what they actually did could be chasmic. Ironically, then, our story begins with texts—the Greek and Roman treatises around which the notion of a Western medical tradition was woven.

KHEIROURGOS

A great deal of Fabricius' practice would have been familiar to his counterparts in the early nineteenth century, but more striking is how much he shared with surgeons working fifteen hundred years before him. *Kheirourgos*, 'hand-worker' in Greek, is the root of the Latin *chirurgus* and the modern English 'surgeon': similarities that go far beyond the name. The notion of a foundational Classical tradition is one of the most potent forces in Western culture, and one that elite Roman practitioners such as Claudius Galen and Cornelius Celsus reworked to encompass their own vision of the clinical art. Most influentially, Galen took the Hippocratic Corpus, a richly polyphonic collection of Greek texts written, mostly, in the fifth and fourth centuries BC, and turned it into a single and powerfully persuasive theory of the body.

In Galen's interpretation—the cornerstone, for more than a thousand years, of elite European and Arabic medicine—health and disease reflected the shifting balance of four humours, governed in turn by the patient's lifestyle and environment. A good physician in the Galenic mould was a skilled observer and a keen listener, familiar with all the failings—physical, mental and moral—to which humanity was prone. He could draw out diagnostic details from the patient's own account of their suffering, and recommend a course of treatment to correct the humoral imbalance underlying these symptoms. For Galen and his contemporaries, there was no necessary opposition between the medical head and the surgical hand.

Surviving Latin texts—Celsus' *De Medicina*, written in the early first century AD, and Galen's second-century *Methodus Medendi*—suggest that any experienced physician would also have had a range of surgical techniques in his repertoire. Mostly these were concerned with the treatment of injuries: splinting fractures, dressing wounds, reducing dislocations, draining abscesses, relieving depressed skull fractures through trepanation, and amputating limbs only if there was no way to preserve their function. This was, in other words, fairly conservative surgery, though Galen—never one to play down his own brilliance or bravery—described cases in which he had successfully repaired the large intestine after a stab wound to the abdomen, or tied off severed arteries through which his patients would otherwise have bled to death. And just as a Galenic physician could also perform skilled surgical interventions, Galenic surgery did not stand in empirical isolation from medical theory.

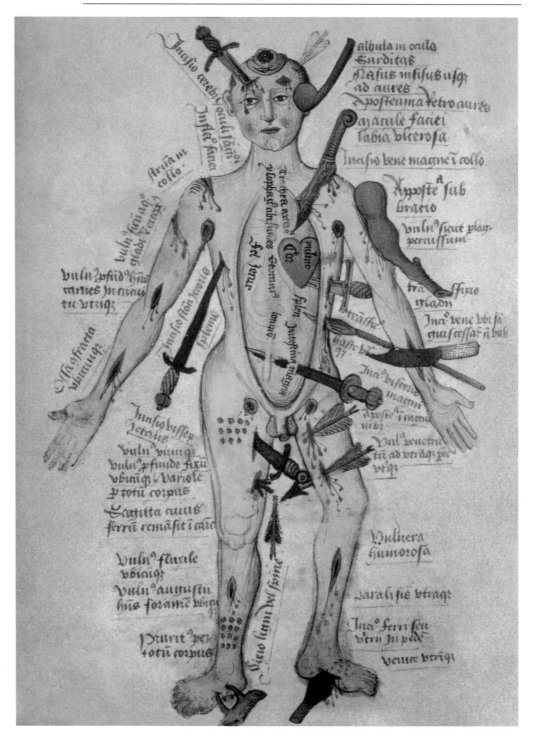

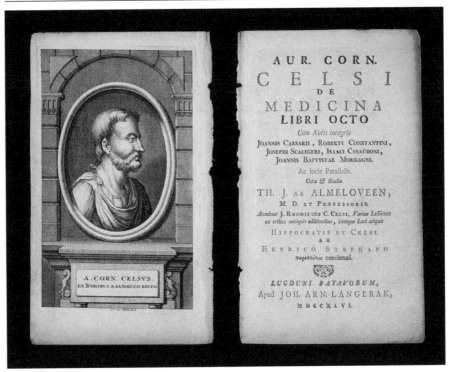

OPPOSITE:
A 'Wound Man', from a fifteenth- or sixteenth-century English anatomical treatise: not, perhaps, a practical guide to human anatomy, but a reminder of the injuries with which a patient might present.

THIS PAGE:
The frontispiece and title page of a 1746 edition of the Roman physician Celsus' writings, featuring an imagined portrait of its author.

Discussing the management of surgical wounds, he argued that blood, the humour of nourishment, was consumed and turned into pus through the process of healing. Certain kinds of suppuration could therefore be taken as a sign that a wound was on the mend.

We know something of what these wealthy and well-respected men wrote about their own practice, how they saw themselves and how they distanced themselves from their rivals; we know much less about what they actually did, and very little about the broader context of Roman medicine and surgery for those who could not afford their expensive attention. Far clearer is their influence on later surgical practice. A chain of what we might call Greco-Latinate whispers connected Celsus and Galen with Arabic physicians of the Islamic Golden Age, French and Italian translators of the high Middle Ages, and early modern scholar-surgeons such as Fabricius. Under the Abbasid caliphate the House of Wisdom in Baghdad became the greatest centre of scholarship in the known world, and physician-philosophers such as Avicenna and Rhazes enriched the Classical tradition with their own research and an Islamic sensibility. New instruments and techniques—a cunning iron guillotine for removing inflamed tonsils, cautery irons for searing wounds and stopping catastrophic blood loss, for example—ran alongside a continued emphasis on conservatism, with a preference for bleeding or cupping patients over amputation or excision.

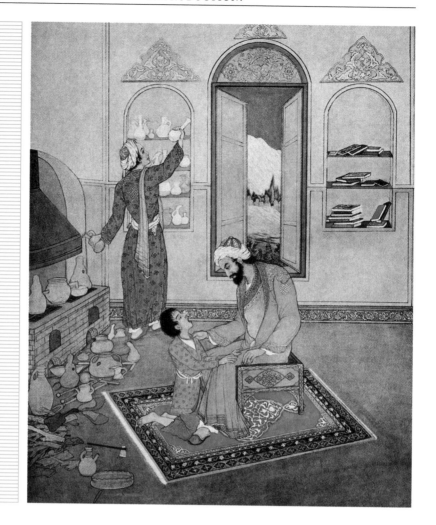

In this print of a painting by the Iranian illustrator Husayn Behzad (1894-1968), the Persian physician Rhazes examines the mouth of a boy in his consulting room, filled with books and alchemical equipment.

What can we surmise about European surgery in the period we still, misleadingly, call the Dark Ages? Medical treatises from the libraries and infirmaries of Benedictine monasteries suggest that monks practised blood-letting and a range of minor surgical interventions. Beyond the gates of God's house, the ninth-century *Leechbook of Bald*—a collection of Saxon medical recipes and instructions—mixed a Classically inflected conservative surgery and a parallel concern for the humoral balance of the body with a form of magical Christianity. We may never know much more about Anglo-Saxon surgery, but another source raises the intriguing possibility that it might not have been quite as painful as we imagine. One twelfth-century English manuscript includes a recipe titled 'How to make a drink that men call dwale to make a man sleep whilst men cut him'. Taken in wine, this compound of hemlock, opium, henbane, lettuce, pig's bile and vinegar also gets a passing mention in Chaucer's 'The Reeve's Tale' (albeit in a context suggesting an aid to sleep, rather than an anaesthetic). Though later surgeons cited dwale only to dismiss it, the name suggests a Scandinavian, perhaps a Viking, origin, and more than fifty recipes survive.

'A LONG ARTE'

I n 1163, the Roman Catholic Council of Tours announced that 'the Church abhors bloodshed'. This was no declaration of mercy for Cathar heretics, then the subjects of a vicious campaign of persecution; ecclesiastical courts would merely hand over condemned prisoners to the secular authorities for execution. But was this statement also, as some have claimed, the origin of the great medieval divide between pious physicians and bloodstained surgeons—the moment when the Classical view of surgery as one strand of learned medicine fell apart? Historians of surgery have been sceptical, arguing that surgery and medicine were pulled apart by broader economic and intellectual currents.

The twelfth and thirteenth centuries witnessed the establishment of many European universities: Paris, Oxford, Cambridge, Bologna and Padua amongst them. Professors of medicine, jostling with philosophers and theologians in the academic hierarchy, increasingly sought to distinguish the learned art of medicine from the merely mechanical art of surgery. Towns and cities, meanwhile, had to find ways of governing the competing trades that operated within their walls. Guilds—fraternities of experienced merchants or craftsmen—were granted monopolies over their business in return for which they trained apprentices and kept order amongst their members. In London, for instance, a Fellowship of Surgeons was established by 1368-9, though by 1435 it had only seventeen members. Surgeons, always more common in towns than educated physicians, also entered guilds with the more numerous barbers (such as London's Company of Barber-Surgeons, formed by merger in 1540). This seemingly odd alliance reflected practical connections: barbers and surgeons both used sharp tools to work on the outside of their customers' bodies.

Here, then, we have a familiar picture of medieval medicine and its hierarchy, with colleges of learned physicians for the wealthy, and urban guilds of barber-surgeons for the middling and lower orders. This is certainly the version of surgical history against which eighteenth- and nineteenth-century surgeons told their stirring tales of progress, but just how accurate is it? Firstly, we might note that this is a largely northern European picture. The more independent, less clerically dominated universities of Italy, Spain and southern France developed their own tradition of 'theoretical surgery' that was quite distinct from the guild practice of German or English barber-surgeons. Informed by the translation of Greco-Roman and Arabic medical treatises, and therefore by the Galenic model of surgery therein, this tradition drew on the same humoral principles as university medicine. It also began to generate its own library of learned writings: the anonymous 'Bamberg surgery', the first known Western surgical treatise, was compiled at the Salerno medical school in southern Italy around 1225.

Even in northern Europe, surviving sources show that the division between physicians and surgeons could be hazy. In England, Bristol and Norwich each established a joint guild of medicine, surgery and barbering, perhaps as a response to the sheer diversity of clinical work in a busy medieval port. In London, meanwhile, Gilbert Kymer—physician to Humphrey, Duke of Gloucester, and eventually chancellor of Oxford University—led a group of surgeons and physicians petitioning the Lord Mayor for a joint college governing all forms of medical practice in London. Though Kymer's college received a charter in 1423, it faded quickly from the historical record, and other cases reveal the ways in which this blurring of professional boundaries could lead to acrimonious disputes over precedence. At the College de St Cosme, founded in Paris in 1210, a faculty of physicians and surgeons oversaw a programme of practical and

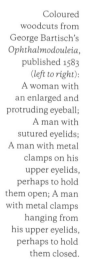

Coloured woodcuts from George Bartisch's *Ophthalmodouleia*, published 1583 (*left to right*): A woman with an enlarged and protruding eyeball; A man with sutured eyelids; A man with metal clamps on his upper eyelids, perhaps to hold them open; A man with metal clamps hanging from his upper eyelids, perhaps to hold them closed.

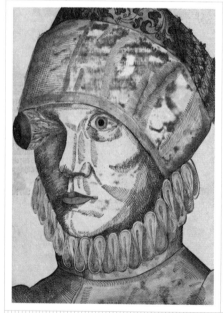
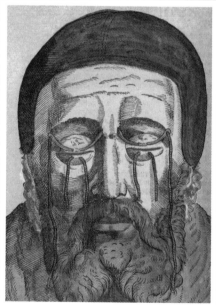

theoretical education, and awarded students three levels of qualification. For the first few centuries of its existence, however, St Cosme was riven by acrimonious quarrels between faculty members and Parisian barbers and surgeons, who became caught up in tensions between students studying for different degrees. Matters came to a head when dissection—overseen by a physician, but actually carried out by a surgeon—entered the curriculum, and it was only in 1516 that this dispute came to an end.

The tensions at St Cosme were resolved in part because physicians and surgeons had found a common enemy: those 'open murtherers' and 'rude empirikes' (in the fighting words of the London surgeon Thomas Gale) who practised medicine and surgery outside the system of colleges and guilds. These unlicensed practitioners were not always as slapdash as Gale's rhetoric suggests—travelling lithotomists or cataract-couchers could be remarkably good (or excruciatingly bad) at their single speciality—but they provided a usefully threatening counterexample against which both surgeons and physicians could advance their claims to professional orthodoxy and authority. Christopher Lawrence and Vivian Nutton have suggested that, by concentrating on the struggles between surgeons and physicians, historians have ignored the ways that leading members of both groups tried to connect their work with the currents of Renaissance humanism. [1] Chaucer's 'Doctour of Physik' could 'speke of physic and of surgerye' (along with astrology and 'magik naturel'), and in his

[1] Christopher Lawrence, 'Democratic, divine and heroic: the history and historiography of surgery', in *Medical Theory, Surgical Practice: Studies in the History of Surgery*, Routledge, 1992, 1-47; Vivian Nutton, 'Humanist surgery', in Andrew Wear *et al* (eds), *The Medical Renaissance of the Sixteenth Century*, Cambridge University Press, 1985, 75-99.

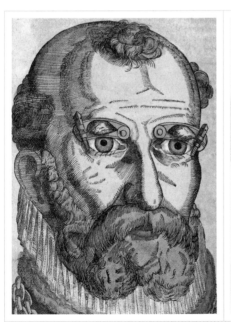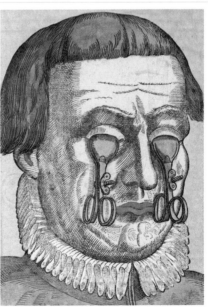

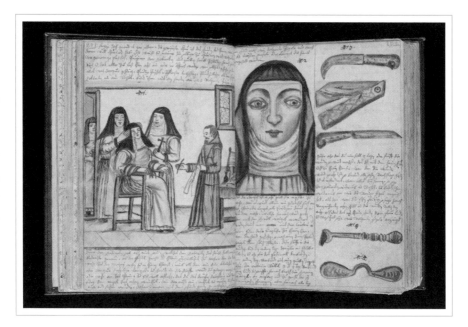

This scene from an *Arzneibuch* (a compendium of surgical techniques and medical recipes), compiled around 1675 for a Franciscan monastery in Germany or Austria, shows surgery for lacrimal fistula being performed on a nun.

Chirurgia Magna, completed in 1363, the French surgeon Guy de Chauliac set out the case for surgery as a humanistic art:

> *The conditions necessary for the surgeon are four: first, he should be learned, second he should be expert: third, he must be ingenious, and fourth, he should be able to adapt himself. It is required for the first that the surgeon should know not only the principles of surgery, but also those of medicine in theory and practice.*

Had not Galen himself regarded medicine and surgery as two halves of a clinically integrated whole? Advocates of humanist surgery took up Galenic debates over wound healing, arguing that 'laudable pus' carried poisoned blood out of the body, and that wounds should not be closed but kept open and allowed to heal 'by second intention' (that is, from the inside out). In 1563, Thomas Gale drew on Classical precedent to make a humanist case for surgery as 'a long arte, [which] requireth longe tyme in lernynge, and also exercising; as both the princes of physicke Hippocrates & Galen do testifie'.

The writings of de Chauliac, Gale and their contemporaries give us a counterintuitive perspective on medieval and early modern surgery, but the notion of humanist surgery had little meaning for patients. Drawing on the southern European tradition of theoretical surgery—often describing operations they admitted they hadn't actually performed or even seen—these

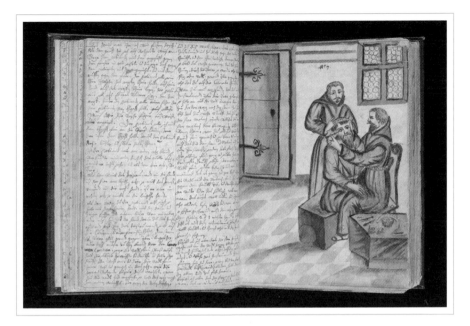

Another
scene from the
Arzneibuch shows
a Franciscan friar
being treated for
cataracts by two
of his fellow friars.

well-read and cultured surgeons gave an exaggeratedly proactive impression of their craft. For most European surgeons, whether northern or southern, as for their predecessors, day-to-day practice was less exciting and more conservative: dressing wounds, letting blood, managing skin diseases. What we have come to see as the set-piece procedures of this kind of surgery—amputation, say, or cutting for the stone—were comparatively rare, performed only when the alternative was chronic pain, permanent incapacity or imminent death.

So what would it have been like to receive treatment from a surgeon in this period? Much would have depended upon a patient's wealth and place of residence: surgeons served as general practitioners for the urban poor and middle orders, and they might treat scurvy, eye diseases or cancer alongside the more usual run of physical injuries. Not all surgical encounters, then, would have been brief and bloody. Patients might stay for a week or more with their surgeon, or take a room in a nearby inn, while he changed the dressings on a wound or repeatedly drained a recalcitrant abscess. The choice of surgeon might also reflect their reputation with a certain technique or tool. Like other craftsmen, surgeons passed expertise or special kit down as family secrets, whether it was the rhinoplasty practised by the Sicilian Branca family, the Chamberlens in London and their obstetrical forceps, or the lateral lithotomy handed down through several generations of the Colot family in France.

Looking through surgical casebooks that survive from the period, we get a vivid impression of the injuries that might have led to a run-in with a

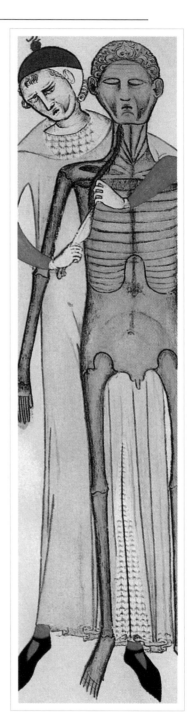

This later facsimile of Mondino de Luzzi's *Anathomia Mundini*, published 1478, shows the dissection of a male cadaver.

surgeon. We read of falls from horses, severe burns from unguarded fires, the appalling damage inflicted by mill machinery and heavy cartwheels, and—the single largest cause of injury in young men—the broken bones, contusions and slashes received in fights, riots and wars. But the barber-surgeon's shop was not the only venue in which these wounds might have been tended. From the twelfth century, hospitals, which were Catholic foundations like the universities, began to appear all over Europe. On the eve of Henry VIII's dissolution of the monasteries, London had perhaps two hundred religious hospitals, some little more than a chapel equipped with beds and staffed by a handful of monks or nuns. Others— such as St Bartholomew's in London, the Hôtel Dieu in Paris, Sta Maria Nuova in Florence—were larger and wealthier, self-contained communities within the cities they served. By the sixteenth century, priests ministering to the souls of inmates worked alongside surgeons taking care of their bodies.

This care was more than just physical. Margaret Pelling argues that, in treating injuries, Tudor barber-surgeons were also helping their customers to refashion themselves in line with a culture that took outward ugliness—particularly damage to the face—as a mark of inner disfigurement.[2] In this sense, barbers and surgeons worked to the same ends: excising a mole or soothing a rash might have a clinical rationale, but it also served the same purpose as trimming a beard or scraping plaque from teeth. City-dwellers found themselves, and their bodies, shaped by new social pressures, and surgery—like fashion, politics or manners—was one way of answering an uncomfortably modern question: how should I present myself to the world?

[2] Margaret Pelling, 'Appearance and reality: barber-surgeons, the body and disease', in A. L. Beier & Roger Findlay (eds), *London 1500–1700: The Making of the Metropolis*, Longman, 1985, 82–112.

THE NEW ANATOMY

I n January 1315, Mondino de Luzzi—professor of anatomy at the University of Bologna, and a leading figure in the southern European tradition of theoretical anatomy—dissected the body of an executed criminal before an audience of medical students. This was not the very first time that a body had been opened for the purposes of medical enquiry. To take just one example, thirteen years earlier a court in Bologna had ordered that the body of one Azzolino be opened, so that a group of physicians and surgeons might find out how he had died. But Mondino's does seem to have been the first public human dissection in Europe for around a thousand years. Over the course of two centuries, Mondino's innovation was taken up first as a way to demonstrate the truths of Classical medicine—and then as a means of overthrowing them.

From the beginning, this style of learning brought physicians and surgeons together. Mondino himself, doubly qualified as a physician and a surgeon, preferred to get his own hands bloody, performing the dissection and explaining the significance of organs and structures to students as he worked. But woodcuts in his *Anatomia Corporis Humani*—written in 1316, first printed in 1478, and one of the standard texts of Renaissance anatomy—show a stylized and hierarchical version of dissection of the sort we've already encountered, with a seated physician reading from a text while a surgeon opened the

LEFT:
Small folding almanacs, such as this one dating from the fifteenth century, gave physicians a portable reference guide to the human body and its astrological connections.

RIGHT:
A Persian 'Zodiac Man', probably twelfth to fourteenth century, showing the association between different parts of the body and the signs of the zodiac.

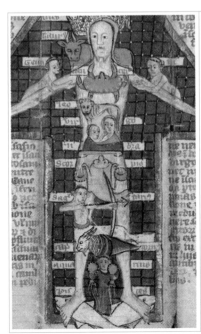

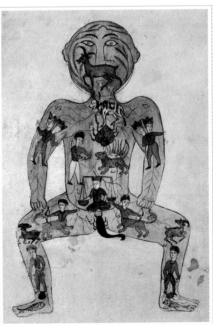

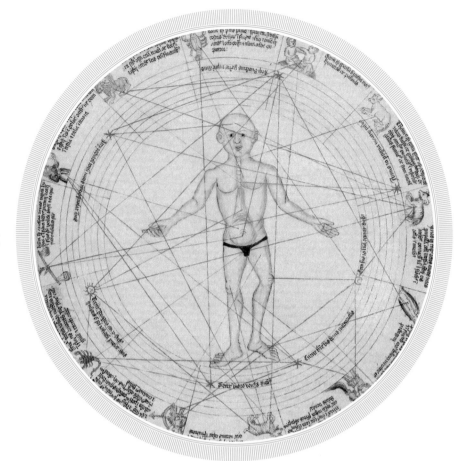

From a German or Bohemian monastic treatise, produced *c.* 1420–1430 and known as the 'Wellcome Apocalypse', this 'Bloodletting Man' shows the influence of planets and constellations on the selection of sites for bloodletting.

body. For Mondino and his learned contemporaries, dissection was a form of philosophical and theological exposition. His *Anatomia* was a practical manual, with human anatomy laid out in the order that a dissection might proceed (with internal organs presented first, before they decomposed beyond recognition). But it also demonstrated the Classical view of human anatomy and the Christian dogma that God had made Man in his own image.

Dissection had been taken up in the medical schools of southern Europe by the end of the fourteenth century, while northern physicians trained in the tradition of theoretical anatomy gradually brought the idea to England and Germany in the fifteenth century. John Caius, a student at the University of Padua and later president of the College of Physicians in London, introduced dissection to his colleagues in London and at Gonville and Caius College in Cambridge. Urban guilds of surgeons also began to hold public dissections: in 1540, Henry VIII granted London's Company of Barber-Surgeons four bodies

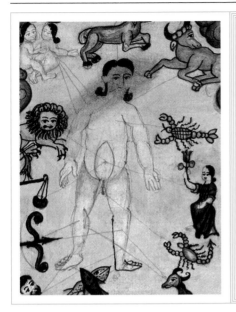

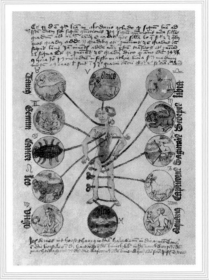

LEFT:
A naked man
surrounded by
the twelve signs
of the zodiac,
from a 1795
Armenian
manuscript.

RIGHT:
A 'Zodiac Man'
from Heymandus
de Veteri Busco's
manuscript *Ars
Computistica*,
written in 1488.

a year from the gallows (and in the following century Charles II made it six). Dissection of the criminal dead was one of several ways in which surgery and medicine were becoming enmeshed in the machinery of state power.

We can see the influence of dissection on European anatomists in the depictions of human bodies that accompanied the anatomical texts they wrote. To modern eyes, this may look like simple progress; illustrations in treatises written at the end of the seventeenth century look much closer to our idea of real human anatomy than those of Mondino's time. What we are actually observing is a shift from schematic and symbolic representations of clinical knowledge—the visual mnemonics of medieval 'Zodiac Men' or 'Wound Men'— to engravings in which surgeons and anatomists tried to capture what they saw when they opened up human bodies. The great emblem of this transformation was *De Humani Corporis Fabrica*, written by Andreas Vesalius, professor of surgery and anatomy at Padua, and published in 1543.

Strange as it may seem, Vesalius—along with other exponents of the New Anatomy of the sixteenth century—was (in Roy Porter's words) 'conservative *in theory*'.[3] Throughout his writings, Galen had insisted that the only way to gain a true appreciation of medicine was not to bury oneself in books but to see for oneself. Vesalius did not set out to overthrow the Classical model of health and disease; instead, he would use Galen's own principles of observation to correct a number of minor errors in Galenic anatomy (caused, he thought, by Galen having dissected only dogs, pigs, apes and sheep). Modern interpretations of the *Fabrica* as a manifesto for scientific surgery have highlighted Vesalius'

[3] Roy Porter, *The Greatest Benefit to Mankind: A Medical History of Humanity from Antiquity to the Present*, Harper Collins, 1997.

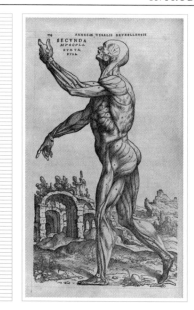

The second in a series of engravings showing human musculature, from Andreas Vesalius' *De Humani Corporis Fabrica*, published 1543.

remarkable gifts as an anatomist, but they have also obscured the question of his influence on his contemporaries.

Thanks in part to magnificently crisp woodcuts thought to have been made by a pupil of Titian, the *Fabrica* was taken up by physicians, surgeons and anatomists reacting against the dominance of Classical medicine. As we have seen, medical colleges and surgical guilds had embraced dissection and practical anatomy in teaching, and some sixteenth- and seventeenth-century surgeons were beginning to commend precise observation as a decisively surgical virtue. The English surgeon Richard Wiseman, drawing on Francis Bacon's influential inductive model of natural philosophy, argued that his colleagues should abandon their book-learning and instead add 'Observations to the bulk of what hath been heretofore heaped up'. His countryman John Halle put it more pithily:

> *A chirurgien should have three diverse properties in his person, that is to say, a heart as the heart of a lion, his eye like the eyes of an hawk, and his hands as the hands of a woman.*

Despite this stirring rhetoric, surgical practice continued much as it had done for centuries. Harvey's demonstration of the circulation of the blood in 1628—later celebrated as a turning point in the history of medicine—changed neither the popularity of therapeutic bloodletting nor the broadly conservative cast of European surgery. Surgeons learned their craft by apprenticeship, organized themselves in guilds, continued to acknowledge their limits as practitioners, and in doing so kept their mortality rates comparatively low. In the notes of the seventeenth-century London surgeon Joseph Binns we find more than 600 cases and 400 recorded outcomes, of which 265 were cured and 62 improved, but only 53 died. Gerhard Eichhorn, a German surgeon who ended his career as *Altamtsmeister* (High Master) of the Cologne barber-surgeons' guild, recorded an even higher rate of success: in his busiest year he treated 200 patients, 95 per cent of whom survived.

Binns' data highlight one way in which surgical practice was changing: his largest single group of patients—almost two hundred—were those suffering from venereal diseases. The treatment of gonorrhoea and syphilis, prevalent in England for a century or more by now, was increasingly seen as the province of surgeons, partly due to their traditional responsibility for the management of skin diseases and partly because of the physical nature of the treatment (involving as it did steam baths, salves and injections of mercury into a patient's urethra). One of the first vernacular treatises on a single disease was the English surgeon William Clowes' 1579 essay on syphilis. Eighteen years later, the Italian Gaspare Tagliacozzi claimed to have perfected a procedure for reconstructing noses eaten away in the late stages of the disease.

But if we were to pick out a single factor behind the emergence of new surgical practices in the sixteenth and seventeenth centuries, the demands of military surgery exercised a far greater influence than the spread of syphilis or even the visual authority of the New Anatomy. Physicians only rarely accompanied armies or navies on expeditions, but surgeons had a recognized and practical role on battlefields and ships, where they dealt with the devastating injuries caused by cannonballs and lead bullets. They also learned how to manage dozens or even hundreds of casualties after a battle, and how to distinguish the critically wounded from those who could wait their turn under the knife.

In the late 1530s, during a campaign in the Italian Wars, the French barber-surgeon Ambroise Paré found that he had run out of the boiling oil widely

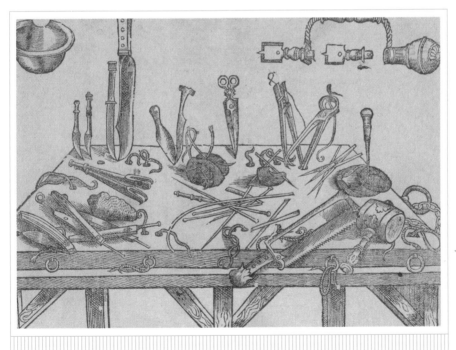

A table of surgical and anatomical instruments, from William Clowes' A Profitable and Necessarie Booke of Observations, for All Those that are Burned with the Flame of Gun-Powder..., published 1637.

The frontispiece
to Thomas
Johnson's English
translation
of Ambroise
Paré's works,
published 1634.

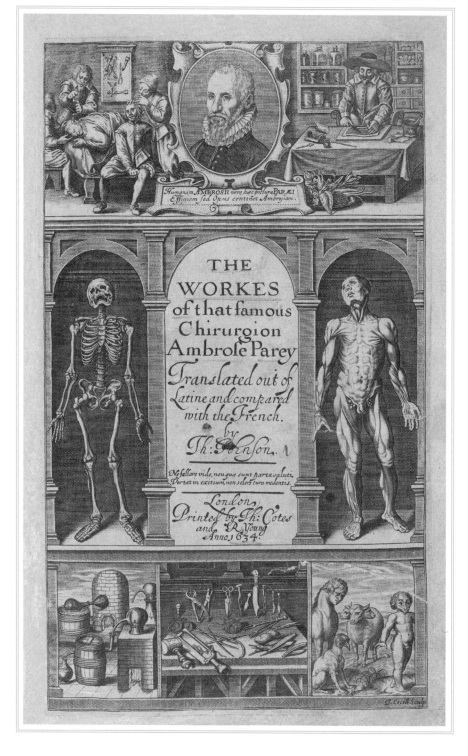

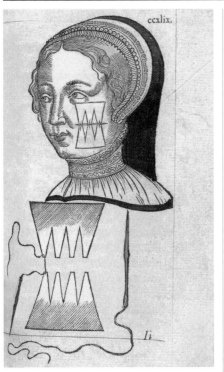

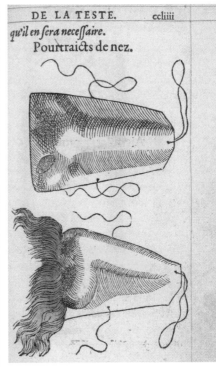

Hand-coloured illustrations from Ambroise Paré's *La Method Curative des Playes, et Fractures de la Teste Humaine*, published 1561:

(*left*) A technique using two pieces of cloth to cure a cheek wound. (*right*) Artificial noses, with or without moustache.

used to cauterize gunshot wounds. Improvising with a salve made from oil of roses, egg white and turpentine, Paré found that wounds dressed in this way gave much less pain and healed more quickly. Paré's position in early modern surgery is tellingly transitional: although he incorporated his own observations into practice and adopted Vesalian anatomy in his publications, he retained Classical ideas of humoral balance in his surgical work.

For English surgeons working in an age of global trade and relentless maritime warfare, naval surgery could be an attractive route to advancement. Joining the navy would give a young surgeon status and regular (though hardly generous) pay, but also a chance to see the world, learn the most demanding surgical practice, and, with hard work and luck, rise through the ranks. English naval surgeons such as John Woodall, Richard Wiseman and William Clowes published practical guides to surgery, and these pocket-sized manuals—written in a hands-on, no-nonsense tone—reflected a new marriage in surgical thought between practical expertise and theoretical reflection.

Hand-coloured
illustrations from
Ambroise Paré's
*Instrumenta
Chyrurgiae et Icones
Anathomicae*,
published 1564:

(*left*) A mechanical
prosthetic hand.
(*right*) A prosthetic
hand made of iron
and attached with
leather straps.

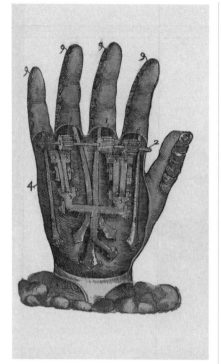

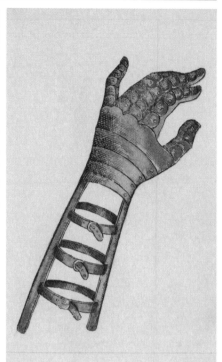

(*left*) A selection
of irons for
cauterizing
wounds. (*right*)
Instruments
and techniques
for extracting
arrows or spears
from wounds.

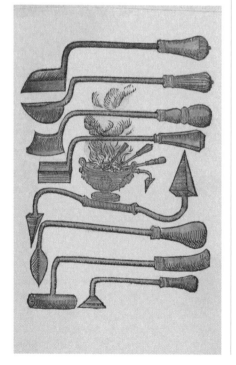

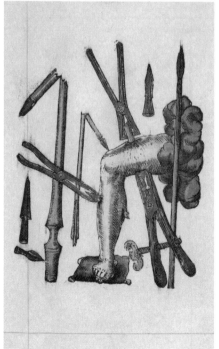

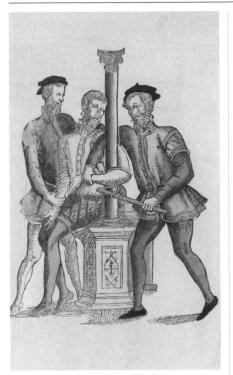

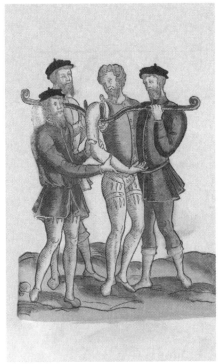

(left) Two surgeons reduce a dislocated elbow. (right) Three surgeons reduce a dislocated shoulder.

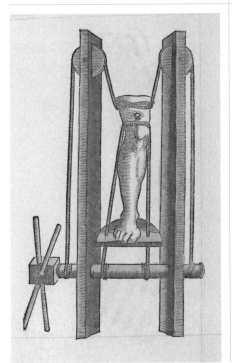

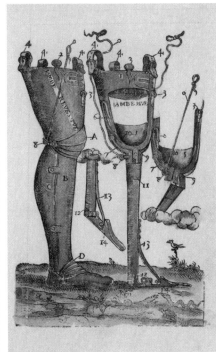

(left) A system of wooden pulleys, possibly for keeping a fractured leg in traction or reducing a dislocated knee. (right) Two wrought-iron prosthetic legs, one made to resemble armour.

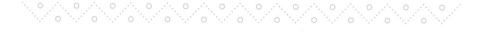

ENLIGHTENED INCISIONS

R esplendent in wig and courtly robes, Guy-Crescent Fagon—premier physician to the Sun King, Louis XIV, and botanist extraordinaire—stood at the peak of early modern learned medicine. As satirists noted, however, even this master of Classical practice was not exempt from the torments of the flesh. By the end of the seventeenth century Fagon was suffering chronic pain from a large bladder stone, and in 1701 he underwent lithotomy with the surgeon Georges Mareschal. Mareschal was himself a highly esteemed practitioner, chief surgeon to the Hôpital de la Charité in Paris, and after the operation he visited his patient to give advice on caring for the wound. 'I needed your hand', Fagon replied loftily, 'but I do not need your head.'

Fagon's retort—a theatrical caricature of the haughty physician, dismissing his surgical servant once the distasteful necessity of surgery was over—might have come straight from a comedy by his near-contemporary Molière. But the Sun King took a different view: he ennobled Mareschal in 1707 and appointed him premier surgeon. Mareschal's rise is a fingerpost to the ways in which surgical theory, identity and ambition would change over the next hundred years. In the spirit of Enlightenment empiricism, looking is an apt metaphor. Surgeons looked back in new ways, rethinking their attitude to the past and rewriting the history of surgery to their own political advantage. They looked forward, making grand predictions of what surgery might achieve as it approached a state of enlightened perfection. They looked away from their traditional craft alliance with the barbers, and towards the professional prestige of the physicians. And they looked inside the human body, seeking to construct a foundation of knowledge from which they might also look up to greater wealth, respect and influence.

Appropriately enough, this movement first emerged in France in the late seventeenth century. In 1672, the French surgeon Pierre Dionis was appointed lecturer in anatomy and surgery at the Jardin du Roi—the medicinal herb garden in which Fagon practised his botany, but also a national centre of clinical teaching. Fifteen years later another surgeon, C.F. Félix, successfully repaired Louis XIV's anal fistula, for which he received the astonishing sum of fifteen thousand gold French sovereigns. Medieval disputes over surgical status at the College of St Cosme were forgotten in 1694 with the construction of a colossal Baroque anatomy theatre, and in 1731 Louis XV extended royal patronage with the foundation of the Académie Royale de Chirurgie. French surgery, though, was not expanding into a vacuum, and leading doctors expressed their opposition to the idea that they should regard surgeons as professional equals in acrimonious 'pamphlet wars'.

During the mid-eighteenth century, the northern and southern European surgical traditions coalesced around this vision of surgery's future. In Paris, the union of barbers and surgeons ended in 1743; two years later, a Company of Surgeons replaced London's medieval guild (and became the Royal College of Surgeons in 1800). The growth of private anatomy schools in the second half of the century—most famously the London school established by William Hunter in 1770—reflected a profound change in the nature of surgical education. An arduous seven-year apprenticeship was no longer the royal road to surgical mastery, and those with enough money might take courses in anatomy or surgery, physiology or zoology, at several different schools, hospitals or museums. European surgery was becoming cosmopolitan, polyglot and interconnected, as students travelled between Edinburgh and Paris, London and Geneva.

Surgical turf wars were not limited to clashes in print with physicians, and from the 1750s surgeons were also encroaching on a traditionally female field of practice. 'Man-midwives' or *accoucheurs*—often, like Hunter or his teacher, the Glaswegian William Smellie, successful and wealthy surgeons—began to cultivate a reputation amongst genteel and aristocratic women, arguing that their detailed grasp of human anatomy gave them an edge over midwives and gossips. By framing their professional competitors as ignorant and old-fashioned, man-midwives could present their own practice as modern and

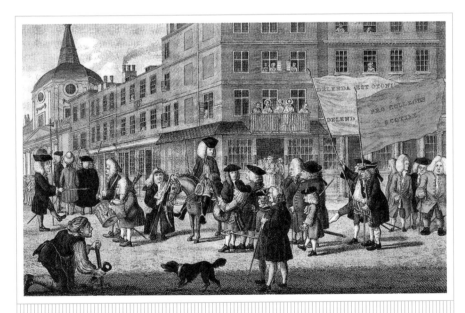

This coloured etching by John June shows licentiates of the Royal College of Physicians marching in protest to the college in 1767.

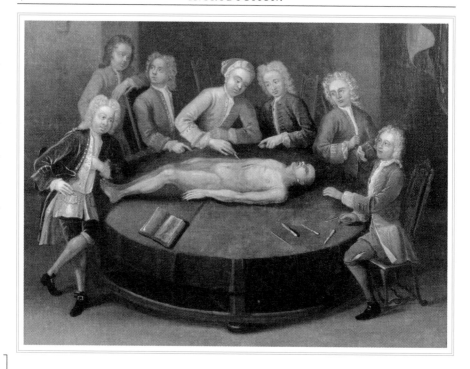

In this oil painting, made around 1730, the anatomist William Cheselden gives an anatomical demonstration to six spectators in the anatomy theatre of the Barber-Surgeons's Company in London.

⁴ Guenter B. Risse, *New Medical Challenges During the Scottish Enlightenment,* Rodopi, 2005.

progressive by contrast, and in so doing carve out a fresh terrain for surgical expertise by—as Guenter B. Risse put it—'medicalizing childbirth, and by extension, all female diseases'.⁴

Surgeons also gained a foothold in eighteenth-century hospitals. Funded by donations and run by committees of local worthies, voluntary hospitals were a standard expression of Enlightenment civic pride, and most appointed at least one surgeon to attend their patients. As the status of these hospitals rose, so did the desirability of a position as a consultant, not least as a way in which an aspiring surgeon could get to know wealthy private clients. Towards the end of the century, London's voluntary hospitals were becoming significant centres of medical education, with theatres for anatomical demonstrations and students accompanying consultants on ward rounds. Surgeons gained a voice in determining admissions in busy casualty wards, and patients—poor and lacking in social capital—provided a source of bodies for dissection if they were unfortunate enough to die under treatment.

Outside hospitals, surgeons were finding greater prospects for employment as European societies responded to industrialization. Wars and colonial expansion meant that naval and military surgeons were still in high demand, and urban asylums, workhouses, jails and dispensaries might all have a resident surgeon on their staff. Barber-surgeons—for centuries the source of basic primary care in northern European towns—were supplanted by a new kind of general practitioner, the surgeon-apothecary. Provincial surgeon-apothecaries might never attain the wealth or fame of William Hunter, but they could expect to live comfortably and respectably, and with a sense that they were participating in the Enlightenment project of 'improvement' through useful knowledge.

What was this useful knowledge on which eighteenth-century surgeons were staking so much? As we might expect, it owed something to the New Anatomy of the sixteenth century, but surgeons also drew on the mechanistic New Philosophy of Descartes, Boyle and Newton. Descartes in particular had analyzed the body as a machine, governed by physical laws, and this, together with the English Royal Society's emphasis on experimentation and personal experience, became the basis of a specifically surgical way of knowing the body. Physicians working with Galenic ideas of health and disease—particularly in the northern European tradition—did not tend to concern themselves with the fine structures of muscular or skeletal anatomy. Their task was to gain a holistic grasp of their patients' lives, not to muddy their minds with useless detail. Taking their cues from Vesalian anatomy, surgeons began to argue that they could build their own independent corpus of knowledge on exactly this sort of precise, attentive anatomical observation.

As with the New Anatomy, this did not go hand in hand with sudden changes in what surgeons actually did. Surgical practice continued to draw on deep roots in craft, with gradual refinements of existing procedures for lithotomy (avoiding damage to the prostate) and the treatment of cataracts (pushing the cloudy lens to one side with a specially designed knife). But anatomo-localism—the idea that the human body in health and disease was best understood in terms of its local physical structure and function—became the dominant dogma of late Enlightenment surgery. And as surgeons such as John Hunter (William's younger brother) began to mix experimentation with dissection and operative practice, they also began to claim that they were the first generation to practise truly 'scientific surgery'.

If surgery was to be accepted as newly scientific it must be seen to have emerged only recently from a barbaric and ignorant past and, in their campaign for a glittering surgical future, eighteenth-century surgeons also rewrote surgery's history. In these new stories, the origins of 'scientific surgery'— rational, humane, independent from medicine—went back no further than a century or two. Those named as its founders—Ambroise Paré in France, William Cheselden or John Hunter in England—were no longer depicted as respectful heirs of Hippocrates or Galen but as insurrectionists, wielding Enlightenment anatomy and physiology against the subservient and unsophisticated prehistory of their discipline. Biographical essays and lectures emphasized character as much as achievement: practitioners of 'scientific surgery' were honourable gentlemen, and as such had as much right to social eminence as physicians.

In aspiring to gentility, surgeons tackled questions that had been exercising physicians for centuries. Traditional codes of genteel deportment were strict and clear: no gentlemen could work with his hands or sell his services for money and, beyond a simple greeting, physical contact—especially between the sexes—was deeply problematic. This created obvious obstacles for any profession concerned with the body, particularly when its members were dependent upon the patronage of wealthy clients. From the seventeenth century, physicians downplayed the practical aspects of medical diagnosis and treatment, concentrating their professional identity around their status as scholars. Eighteenth-century surgeons took a different tack, making manual skill the core of their identity, but also using the rhetoric of 'scientific surgery' to argue that this was an entirely appropriate pursuit for an Enlightenment gentleman. Physicians might present themselves as grave, lean and learned; in portraits and caricatures surgeons were more robust, with an air of worldly empiricism that was coming to serve them well. According to John Gregory, professor of the practice of medicine at Edinburgh, writing in 1772:

> If a surgeon or apothecary has had the education and acquired the knowledge of a physician, he is a physician to all intents and purposes... and ought to be respected and treated accordingly.

By the end of the eighteenth century leading surgeons had achieved professional parity, more or less, with physicians. It was in the hospitals of the French Revolution that this equality acquired a radical cast.

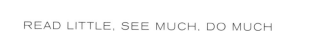

READ LITTLE, SEE MUCH, DO MUCH

A s a sequence of historical events, the story of 'Paris medicine' is easily told. Within a year of the storming of the Bastille in July 1789, the new National Constituent Assembly abolished monastic vows and dissolved religious orders in an assault on the institutions of the *ancien regime*. By doing so, it also closed down the majority of French hospitals. By 1794, the Revolutionary Council had ordered a reorganization of medical education, partly in response to the pressing need for military surgeons as other European nations declared war on France. Large urban infirmaries were renamed—in Paris the Hôtel Dieu became the Hospice d'Humanité—

and reopened as secular, state-funded teaching hospitals. Under this new dispensation, medical and surgical students worked alongside one another, receiving the same basic education in anatomy and physiology and gaining first-hand experience of the physical basis of disease by dissecting the bodies of patients who died on the wards. Students from all over Europe and the United States came to study in these hospitals, and within a generation Paris medicine had become the dominant Western model of medical education.

Understanding the significance of these events, though, is less straight-forward, and for almost a century scholars have disagreed profoundly over their meaning and nature. Does Paris medicine represent the culmination of trends that had been developing gradually in Europe for a century or more, or should we understand it as a rupture in the social and intellectual fabric of medicine? Owsei Temkin, one of the earliest and most influential historians of Paris medicine, argued that it was the moment in which medicine acquired 'the surgical point of view'—the tradition of empirical anatomo-localist thinking that had emerged in European surgery over the eighteenth century.[5] The Parisian physician Pierre Cabanis may have urged his students to 'read little, see much, do much', but (as Temkin noted) surgeons had been working in this way for hundreds of years. In the hospitals of Paris the interior of the body became, at least in principle, a domain of surgical theory and practice, while surgery itself became a paradigm of localized curative intervention—a model for what medicine might achieve in the nineteenth century.

Following Temkin's line of argument, there are ways in which Paris medicine looks like the outcome of more gradual currents of change. From the middle of the eighteenth century medical and surgical students had shared classes at private anatomy schools, and hospitals in cities such as Edinburgh were becoming important centres of surgical teaching and practice well before 1794. Some historians have argued that the most significant distinction in European medicine on the eve of the French Revolution was not between surgeons and physicians, but between the work of hospital consultants and the community practice of surgeon-apothecaries. Intellectually, too, we can trace what seems to be a clear thread from the 'solidist' physiology of the Swiss anatomist Albrecht von Haller, via the classic Enlightenment anatomo-localism expressed in Giovanni Battista Morgagni's *De Sedibus et Causis Morborum*, published in 1761, to Xavier Bichat's tissue pathology, developed at the Hôtel Dieu in the late 1790s.

For the historian and philosopher Michel Foucault, this line of gradual descent was an illusion.[6] Foucault figured Paris medicine as a discontinuity in the relationship between knowledge and power, in which 'anatomopolitics' figures as one of several tools for policing the citizens of industrial societies. Against Temkin's gradualism, he also argued that eighteenth-century anatomo-localism differed fundamentally from the ideas underpinning Paris medicine.

[5] Owsei Temkin, 'The role of surgery in the rise of modern medical thought', *Bulletin of the History of Medicine* 25, 1951, 248-259.

[6] Michel Foucault, *The Birth of the Clinic: An Archaeology of Medical Perception* [1963], trans. Alan Sheridan, Tavistock, 1973.

Morgagni, for example, constructed pathological taxonomies in which all diseases afflicting (say) the chest were related and, following the precedent of Classical humoralism, might move around the body to afflict other organs. For Bichat, however, the physical structure of particular tissues made diseases highly specific; asthma would no more afflict the joints of the big toe than gout would migrate to the lungs.

For our purposes, one strand of Temkin's argument remains compelling. If disease were the result not of generalized humoral imbalances but of localized physical lesions—tumours, abscesses, malformations—then under the regime of Paris medicine these lesions became uniquely amenable to surgical treatment. Aspects of the old consensus died hard. Using statistical data from hospital records, Parisian physicians spent almost a generation arguing over the therapeutic value of bloodletting, and musing on the fact that hardly anything they did actually cured their patients. Critics called Paris medicine morbid, obsessed with disease and death at the expense of understanding life and health. But for European surgeons, Paris medicine put 'the surgical point of view' at the heart of early nineteenth-century medical thinking.

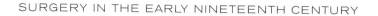

SURGERY IN THE EARLY NINETEENTH CENTURY

S urgeons who came of age in the era of Paris medicine found it easy to believe—and not without reason—that they were living at the end of one century of surgical upheaval rather than at the beginning of another. Most of the aspirations expressed by Enlightenment surgeons had been achieved: surgery was widely recognized as a profession, with national institutions and the hospital as a citadel of authority. A generation of virtuoso surgical celebrities trod the boards in London's operating theatres: the suave Astley Cooper, who received a baronetcy for removing a cyst from the scalp of George IV, and who earned £15,000 (in today's terms, more than £1 million / $1.5 million) a year at the height of his fame; the fierce Robert Liston, who operated with a knife gripped between his teeth, and who could amputate

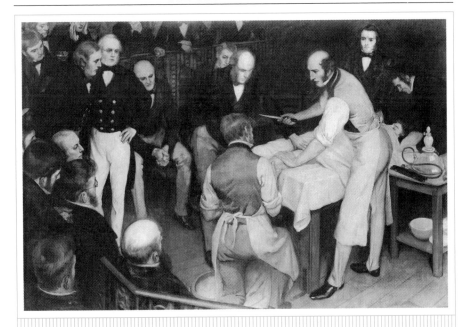

Commissioned by Henry Wellcome and made in 1912 by Ernest Board, this painting reconstructs one of the first British operations carried out with anaesthesia by the surgeon Robert Liston.

a leg in under three minutes. As Temkin pointed out, 'surgery, with all its imperfections before 1846, could and did cure with some confidence'.[7]

[7] Temkin, 1951.

From the perspective of the early twenty-first century, though, things look rather different. Operations were still conducted as swiftly as possible, with no pain relief for patients and comparatively high rates of death from post-operative infections. But the history of surgery in the nineteenth century is—as the following essays show—far more than the challenge of finding technical solutions to two pressing clinical problems. Stale questions demanded fresh answers. How should surgeons work with physicians, and vice versa? Which was more important, theoretical understanding or practical finesse? How would ideas such as germ theory affect surgery's status and independence? In the encounter between clinician and patient, who should have the last word in determining the course of action? What were the limits (if any existed) to surgery's curative power?

To these questions we can add a few of our own contemporary concerns. How did cultural, economic and intellectual developments affect what went on in operating theatres? Why did the role of women in operating theatres begin to change? Most importantly, what did all this mean for patients? To find the answers to these questions, we'll follow the story of surgery through its most remarkable century of revolution.

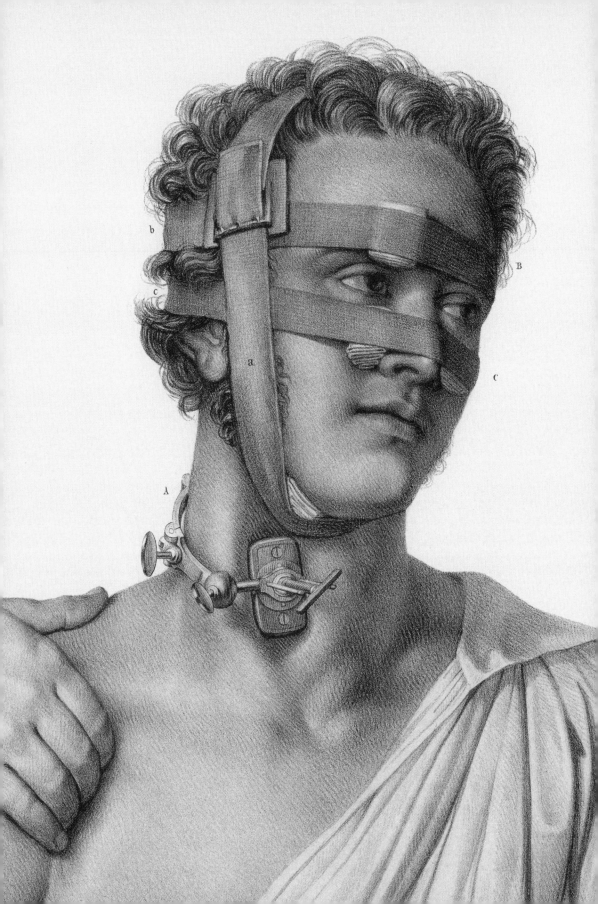

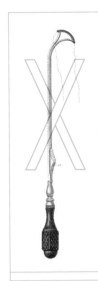

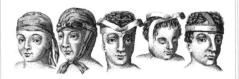

HEAD & NECK

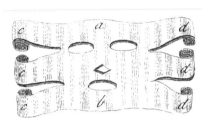

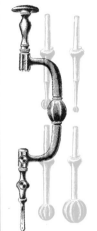

HEAD.

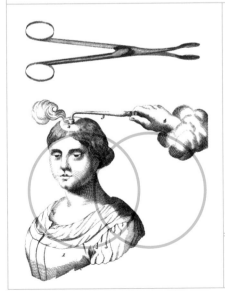

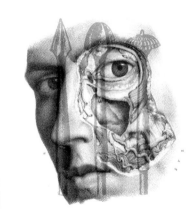

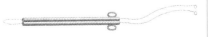

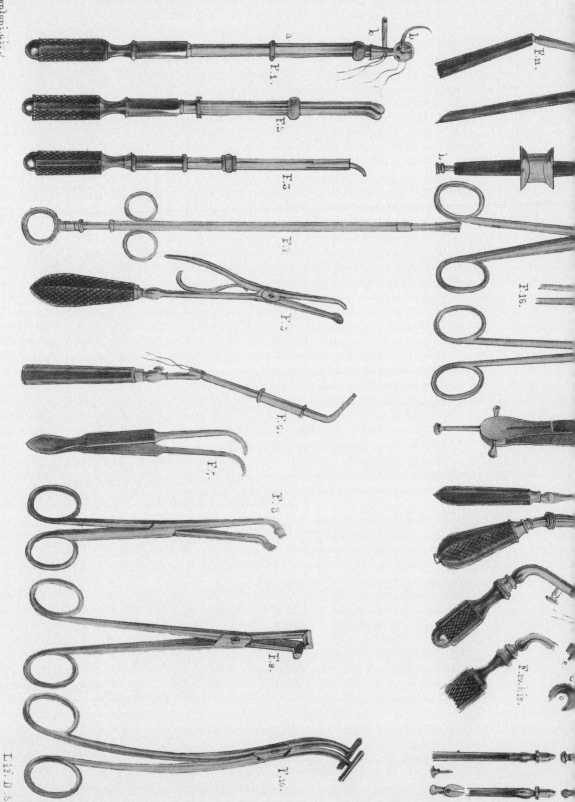

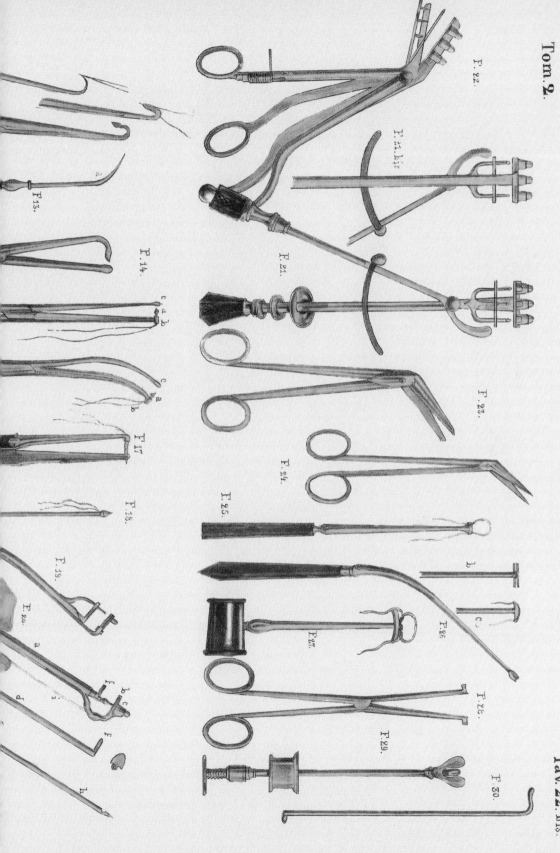

Tom. 2.

F. 22.
F. 21. bis
F. 21.
F. 13.
F. 14.
F. 17
F. 23.
F. 24.
F. 25.
F. 18.
F. 19.
F. 20.
F. 26.
F. 27.
F. 28.
F. 29.
F. 30.

Tav. 22. bis.

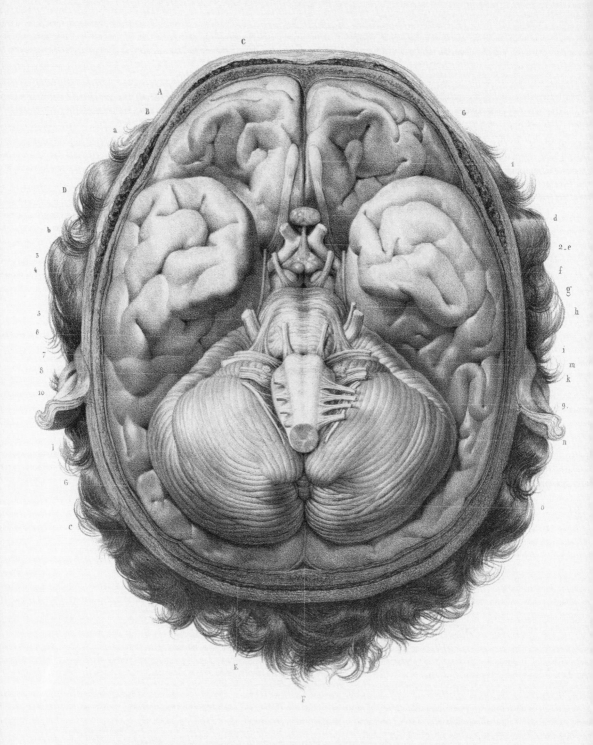

PREVIOUS: PAGE 46 | A method of stemming bleeding from the carotid and axillary arteries of the head and neck, using straps, pads, and a compression clamp to apply pressure. PAGES 48-49 | Instruments used to correct cleft palates.

ABOVE: Anatomy of the human brain seen from below, showing the brain stem, cerebellum, and roots of the cranial nerves.

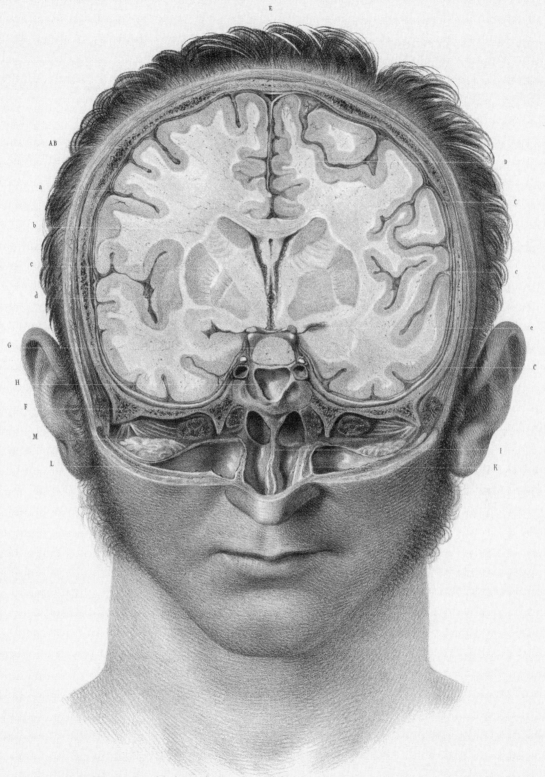

ABOVE: Vertical cross section of the human brain.

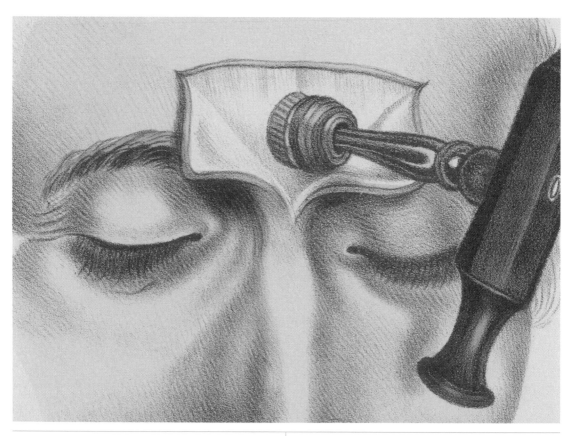

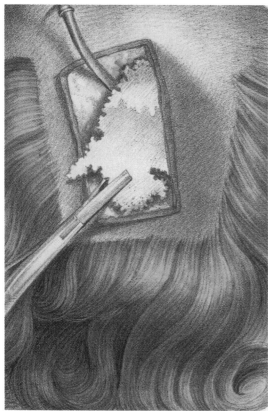

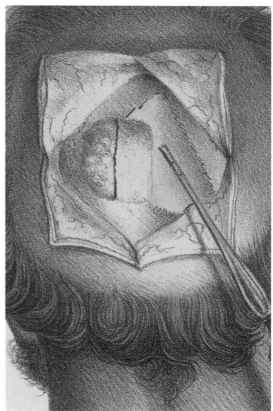

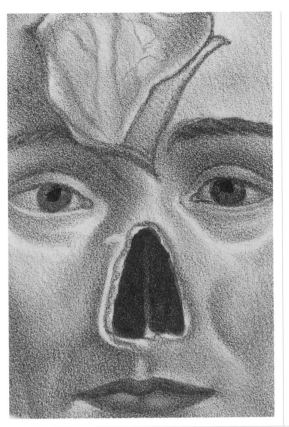
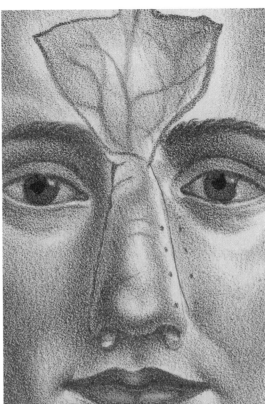
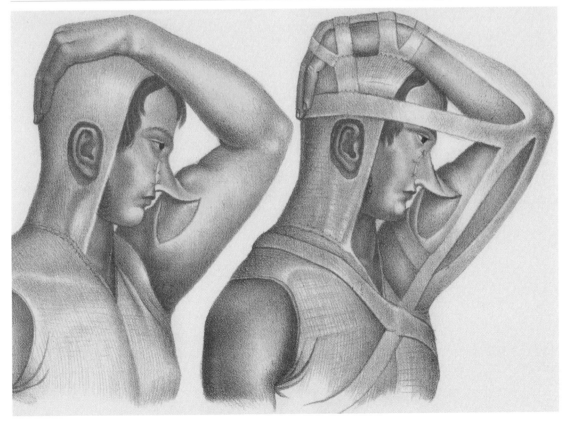

PREVIOUS: PAGE 52 *(top)* Perforation of the frontal sinuses using a hand-powered circular saw. *(bottom left)* Removal of a piece of inflamed skull, using forceps and levers. *(bottom right)* Removal of a wedge of skull, using a small triangular saw. PAGE 53 *(top left)* First stage of rhinoplasty (surgery to reconstruct the nose), using a flap of forehead skin. *(top right)* Second stage of rhinoplasty, using a flap of forehead skin. *(bottom)* Rhinoplasty using a flap of skin from the upper arm.

THIS PAGE & OPPOSITE: Techniques for repairing various kinds of harelip.

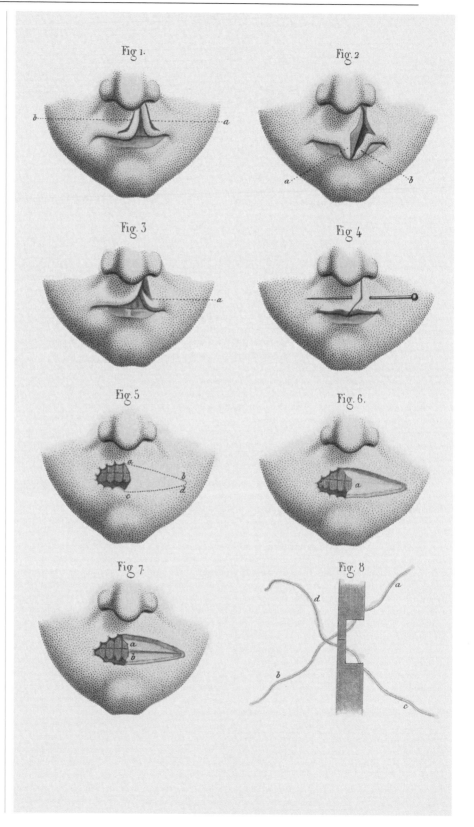

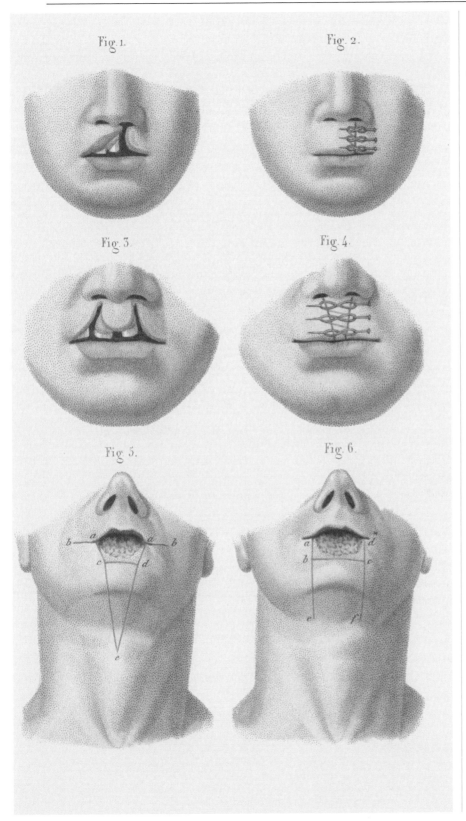

Fig. 1.

Fig. 2.

Fig. 3.

Fig. 4.

Fig. 5.

Fig. 6.

OVERLEAF:
PAGE 56-57 | Techniques
for repairing injuries to
the cheeks, lips and chin.
PAGE 58 | Resection of
the upper jaw. PAGE 59 |
Resection of the lower jaw.

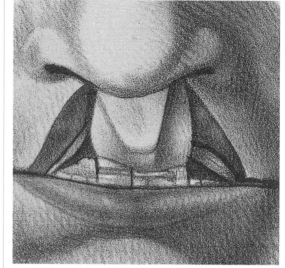

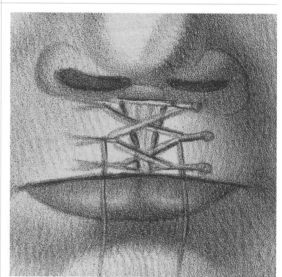

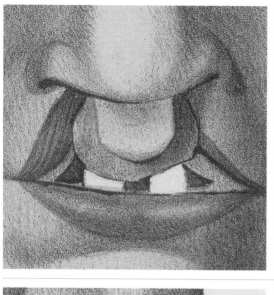

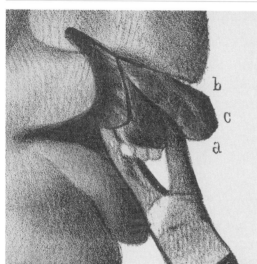

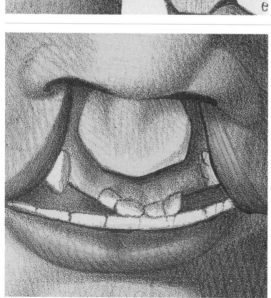

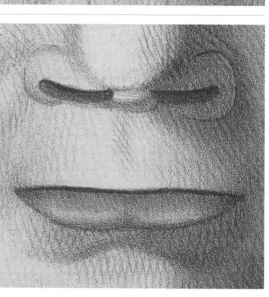

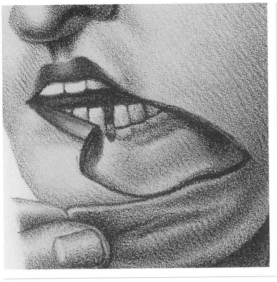
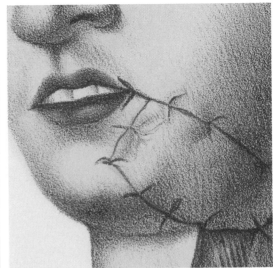
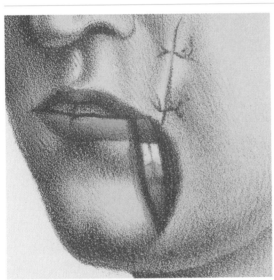
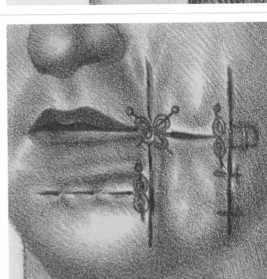
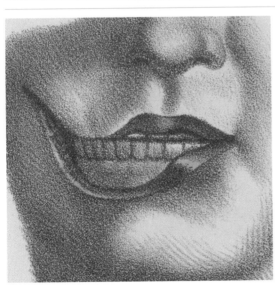
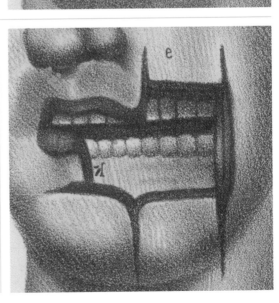

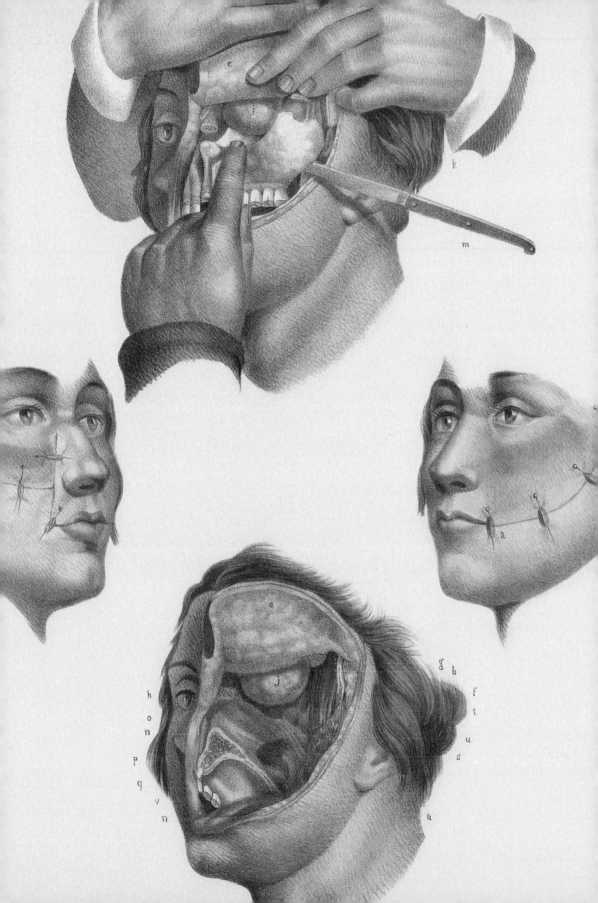

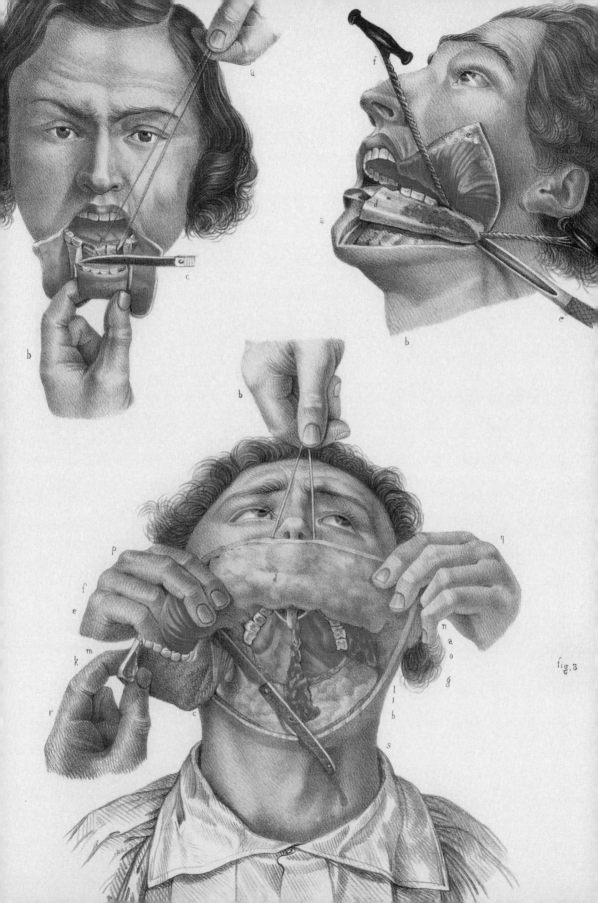

fig.3

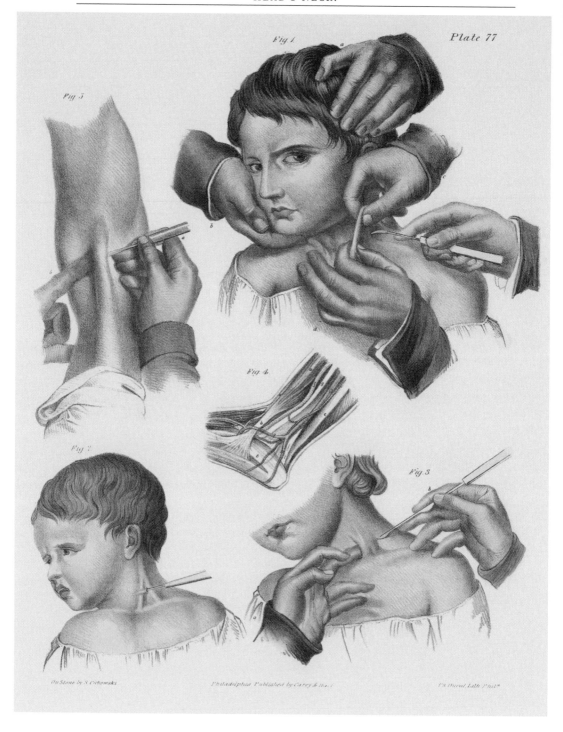

ABOVE: Various operations carried out through a small opening in the skin.
OPPOSITE: Surgical incisions in the jugular and cephalic arteries.

Plate 4

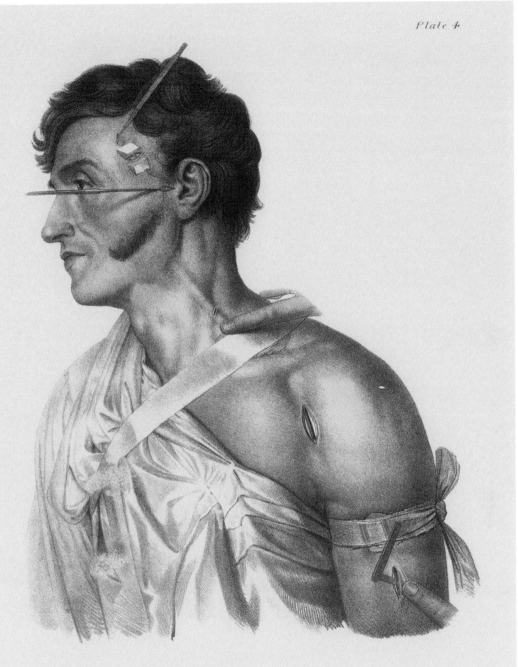

In Stone by Newsam   Philadelphia. Published by Carey & Hart   P.S. Duval, Lith. Phila.

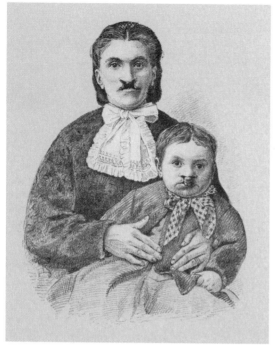
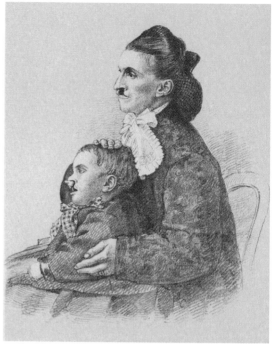
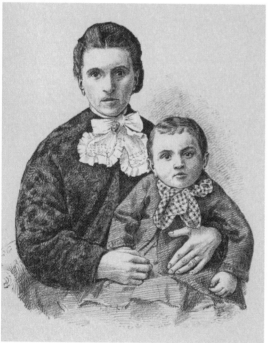
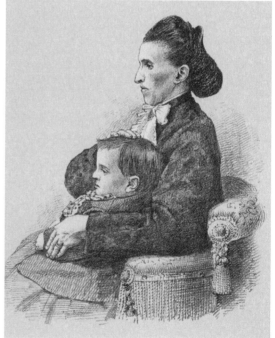

ABOVE: Double complicated harelip in mother and child. Front and side views before (*top*) and after (*bottom*) surgery.
OPPOSITE: Enormous fibro-cellular tumour. Front and side views before (*top*) and after (*bottom*) surgery.

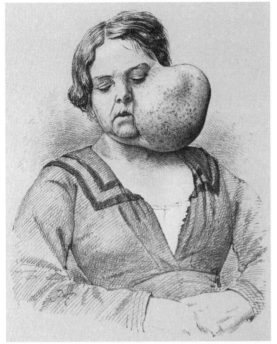

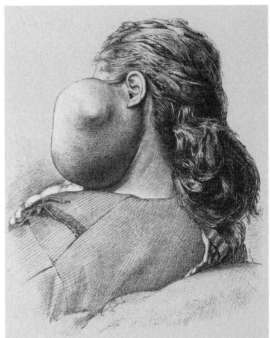

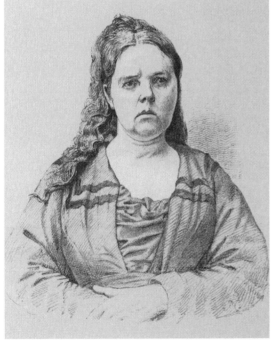

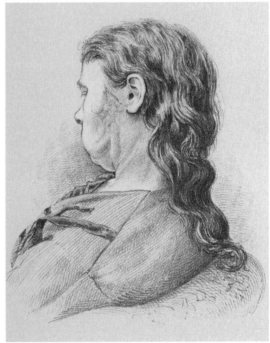

THE YANKEE DODGE: *Anaesthesia.*

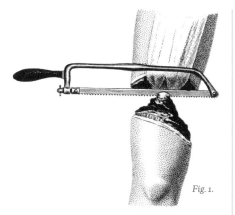

Fig. 1.

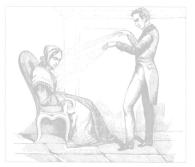

Fig. 2.

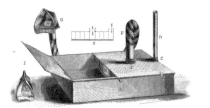

Fig. 3.

In November 1842, W. Squire Ward, surgeon to the Ollerton Infirmary near Nottingham, cut off the leg of one J. Wombell, a forty-two-year-old labourer. This was no ordinary amputation: Ward's assistant, the Middle Temple barrister William Topham, was experimenting with a radical new technique for rendering patients insensible and making surgery painless. Wombell moaned once or twice during the surgery but remained unconscious, and afterwards declared that he had felt no pain whatsoever.

Topham's technique was not anaesthesia but mesmerism, and the first widely acknowledged painless operation is usually said to have taken place four years later, when the American dentist William Morton administered ether to a patient at the Massachusetts General Hospital on 16 October 1846. By the end of the nineteenth century surgeons were marking this date—not that of Wombell's operation—as a crowning moment of scientific and humanitarian progress. But the story of Ward, Topham and Wombell raises other questions we might want to ask. If physicians and natural philosophers had been experimenting with gases such as nitrous oxide as far back as the 1790s, why did anaesthesia not emerge for a generation or more? Why did a few surgeons regard mesmerism, rather than chemically induced unconsciousness, as the greatest hope for painless surgery? Why did some patients and practitioners initially resist the offer of painless surgery?

We might think that before 1846 surgeons were heartily and necessarily indifferent to the agonies of their patients. Indeed, the phrenologist Johann Gaspar Spurzheim argued that the brains of surgeons tended to exhibit large 'Organs of Destructiveness', enabling them to inflict pain on others without compunction. In diaries, letters and memoirs, eighteenth- and nineteenth-century practitioners expressed intense ambivalence about the suffering they inflicted. Equally, though, the same sources demonstrate that surgeons' anxieties over inflicting pain did not stop them pushing at the accepted limits of surgical practice. In the decades preceding Morton's 1846 operation under ether, surgeons, especially those in the United States, were developing 'a range of complicated operations, many of which required a protracted period at the operating bench'.[1] By the 1840s, Paris medicine had already rewritten the scope and goals of surgery; anaesthesia made this acceptable to patients and to the public.

Anaesthesia in its modern sense—controllable, reversible, administered through inhalation—has its foundations in the work of a handful of politically and intellectually adventurous chemists in the late eighteenth century. Joseph Priestley seems to have been the first to prepare nitrous oxide in 1772, and by 1795 the young Humphry Davy was experimenting with it at Thomas Beddoes' Pneumatic Institute in Bristol. Five years later he wrote that inhalations of nitrous oxide had relieved the pain of a bad tooth, and that it 'may probably be used with advantage during surgical operations'. So why was it not taken up immediately as an anaesthetic? Partly this was down to what Davy was trying to achieve. The Pneumatic Institute had been established to find new treatments for consumption, which Beddoes and Davy understood (in accordance with the Scottish physician John Brown's theories of nervous excitation) as a lack of bodily stimulation. For them, nitrous oxide was not an exciting new anaesthetic but an unsuccessful

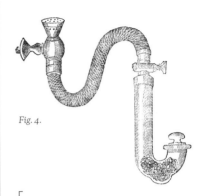

Fig. 4.

[1] Christopher Lawrence, 'Democratic, divine and heroic: the history and historiography of surgery', in *Medical Theory, Surgical Practice: Studies in the History of Surgery*, Routledge, 1992, 1-47.

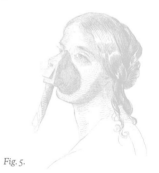

Fig. 5.

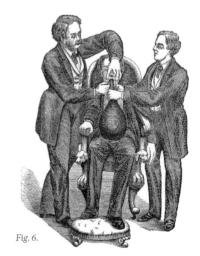

Fig. 6.

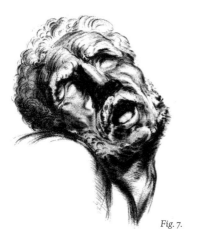

Fig. 7.

[2] Alison Winter, *Mesmerised: Powers of Mind in Victorian Britain*, University of Chicago Press, 1998.

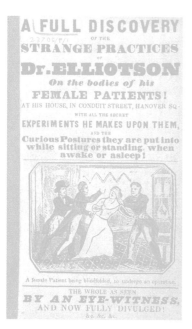

Fig. 8.

treatment for consumption. More than this, it produced wildly different effects in those who inhaled it; perhaps its power of numbing pain might depend on the character and sensibility of individual patients?

Clinical and cultural attitudes to pain at this time were intensely ambivalent. Older ideas of pain as a trial from God, to be suffered penitently, even gratefully, and not dodged with drugs, were only gradually fading under the influence of the Enlightenment's emphasis on humane improvement. Surgeons knew the pain of surgery could be daunting, but was it necessary for surgical success? By maintaining and sharpening consciousness, they thought it helped patients to survive operations, and induced essential healing processes. In a pamphlet published in 1824 Henry Hill Hickman, a Shropshire surgeon, described operations on animals after knocking them out with carbon dioxide. But for most surgeons, carbon dioxide, nitrous oxide or older drugs such as laudanum only seemed to bring patients closer to death—exactly what they fought so hard to avert.

Alison Winter has observed the curious parallels between the development of early anaesthetics such as nitrous oxide and ether, and the emergence of mesmerism. [2] Both first appeared in the hands of late Enlightenment political radicals; in the early nineteenth century both became staples of travelling variety shows in Europe and the United States; and both induced a troubling state of 'suspended sensibility'. In Britain the most prominent medical proponent of mesmerism was John Elliotson, professor of medicine at University College London from 1832. Elliotson gained support from his circle of literary friends, which included Thackeray, Dickens and Wilkie Collins, but in 1838 he was forced from his professorship after a scandal over what the *Lancet* claimed were fraudulent demonstrations of mesmerism by his protégées, the O'Key sisters. Four years later James Braid, a Scottish surgeon working in Manchester, began to use a

stripped-down version of mesmerism—hypnotism—
in his practice. Braid abandoned the more
extravagant claims of the mesmerists (particularly
the notion that they generated their effects by
manipulating streams of magnetic subtle fluids),
but by the end of the decade interest in his work
had been swept away by the success of anaesthesia.

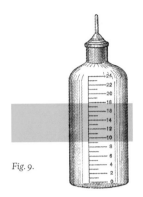

Watching 'ether frolics' at country fairs in the
1830s and early 1840s, several American dentists
and doctors had the same thought, and began to
pull teeth or remove small cysts from patients under
the influence of ether or nitrous oxide. Theirs is
as much a story of commercial opportunism as of
heroic humanitarianism, and quarrels over patents
and priority continued decades after their deaths.

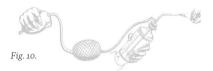

Fig. 9.

Word spread rapidly after Morton's demonstration
at the Massachusetts General, and on 19 December
1846 the dentist James Robinson—so nervous that
his glass inhaler shook in his hands—gave the first
British general anaesthetic to a patient at University
College Hospital in London. After conducting a
mid-thigh amputation without a sound from his
patient, the Scottish surgeon Robert Liston turned
to his audience and said 'This Yankee dodge,
gentlemen, beats mesmerism hollow.'

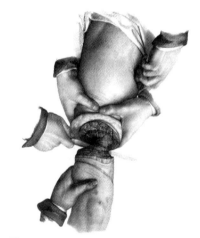

Fig. 10.

Responses to this innovation were not as
straightforward as one might expect. For the first
generation of anaesthetists—dentists or general
practitioners who took up anaesthetics as a
sideline—the major technical problem was dosage.
Administering ether through a simple bellows
inhaler, or even on a silk handkerchief pressed to
the nose, they found it fatally easy to overdose and
kill their patients. In 1847 John Snow (now better
known for his work on the transmission of cholera)
applied John Dalton's gas physics to the design of
an ether inhaler that would regulate dosage, and
also enable patients to start breathing the irritating
vapour gradually. Even when given in lower
concentrations, ether could produce alarming
effects: consumptive patients turned purple, while
others bled freely when the first incision was made.

Fig. 11.

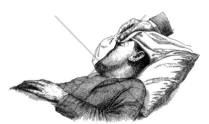

Fig. 12.

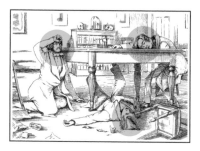

Fig. 13.

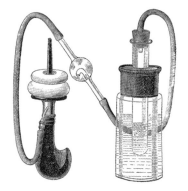

Fig. 14.

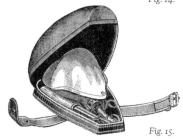

Fig. 15.

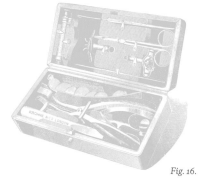

Fig. 16.

James Young Simpson, an Edinburgh surgeon and obstetrician, found that another volatile liquid was equally effective and far more pleasant to breathe. In the late 1840s, though, a series of deaths showed that chloroform could kill quickly and without warning by affecting the action of the heart. Nineteenth-century anaesthesia thus tended to be kept shallow, with patients talking (and even singing) as the surgeon set to work. This brought its own problems: under light anaesthesia muscles could be squirmy or stiff, and inhalers got in the way of operations on the face, mouth and neck. One solution was local anaesthesia, pioneered in Vienna by the eye surgeon Carl Koller. His colleague Sigmund Freud, then a young neurologist, had noted the numbing effects of a cocaine solution, and Koller found that injections could be used to block nerves or infiltrate spinal fluid.

This strangely ambiguous new state of consciousness evoked characteristically Victorian anxieties. Snow and Simpson argued that anyone fit for surgery was fit for anaesthesia, but in its first decade most surgeons reserved it for patients at the lowest risk of death or those—women, children—thought to be least resistant to pain. Some questioned whether anaesthesia might make soldiers and sailors more susceptible to pain, and hence less fearless in battle. Would surgeons operate less carefully if their patients were no longer conscious? Would outwardly respectable folk become madmen or nymphomaniacs as they began to breathe the gas? As early as 1849, newspapers were alarming their readers with reports of gangs using chloroform to rob or kidnap victims. Within two decades, anaesthesia was accepted across Europe and the United States, but these concerns show that nineteenth-century surgery relied heavily on trust—between individual patients and surgeons, between the profession and the public.

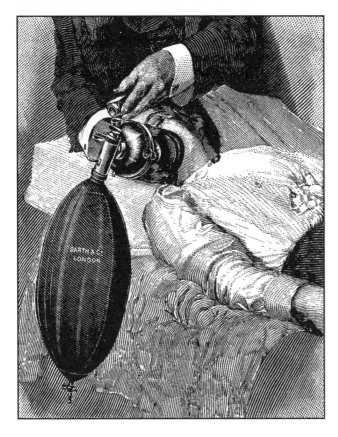

Fig. 17.

FIG. 1: *This engraving made in 1844, just before the advent of anaesthesia, gives some sense of the technical challenges of amputation—but no indication of the pain it inflicted.* FIG. 2: *Early mesmerists believed they could cure disease and alter states of mind by manipulating rays of 'animal magnetism', as in this 1845 woodcut.* FIG. 3: *Regulating dosage was a major problem for early anaesthetists. This ether inhaler, designed by London anaesthetist and GP John Snow (1813-1858) in 1847, used a bath of warm water to minimize fluctuations in the concentration of ether vapour.* FIG. 4: *Many physicians designed and built their own anaesthetic inhalers—such as this one from 1847.* FIG. 5: *Masks such as this one, designed by John Snow in 1847, gradually replaced cumbersome and inefficient glass ether inhalers.* FIG. 6: *American dentists had used nitrous oxide as a short-acting anaesthetic since the late 1830s, usually administering it in bladders or (as shown here) balloons.* FIG. 7: *Early modern surgeons would have been intimately familiar with the kind of agony depicted in this portrait from the anatomist Charles Bell's* The Anatomy and Philosophy of Expression, *1844.* FIG. 8: *John Elliotson's (1791-1868) experiments with mesmerism provoked controversy and sensationalism, as in this lurid 1842 pamphlet.* FIG. 9: *Chloroform was easier to administer than ether and could be shaken from a drop bottle onto a handkerchief.* FIG. 10: *Country doctors, travelling long distances from patient to patient, favoured small portable ether inhalers such as this one.* FIG. 11: *With anaesthesia, major amputations—here a circular amputation of the leg above the knee—became slower, calmer and quieter affairs.* FIG. 12: *Even after the development of inhalers, the leading surgeon Joseph Lister (1827-1912) preferred to administer chloroform on the corner of a towel placed over the patient's mouth.* FIG. 13: *James Young Simpson (1811-1870) claimed to have discovered the properties of chloroform after drinking a glass with two friends after a dinner party.* FIG. 14: *For patients with severe facial injuries, or those who could not tolerate a mask, ether could be administered via the rectum.* FIG. 15: *Nineteenth-century anaesthetic equipment tended to be small and simple, such as this chloroform inhaler set.* FIG. 16: *Surgeons working in remote areas or on board ship carried small sets of instruments, such as this one, to administer anaesthesia while carrying out emergency surgery.* FIG. 17: *In the early twentieth century, anaesthetic equipment grew larger and more sophisticated—witness this nitrous oxide inhaler from 1922— and anaesthesia became a clinical speciality.*

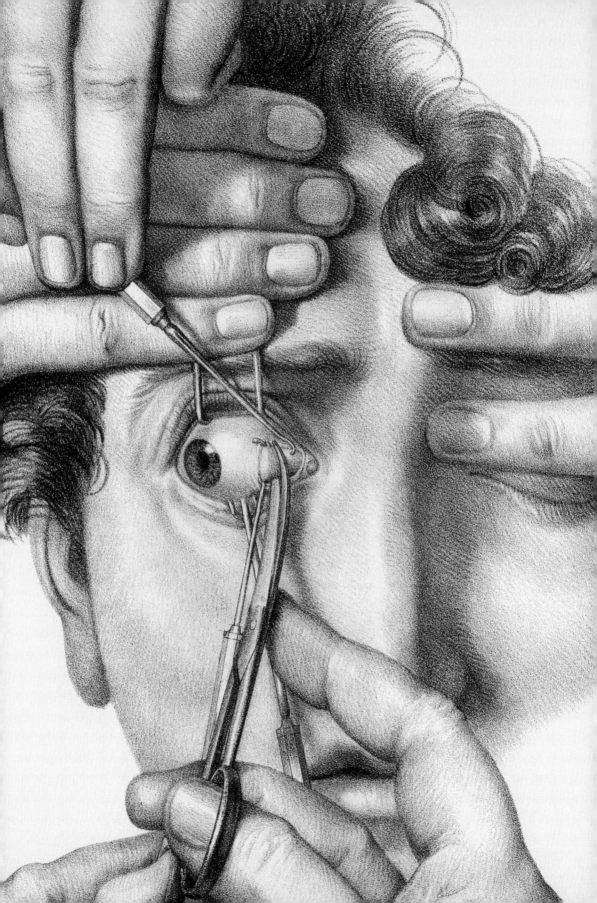

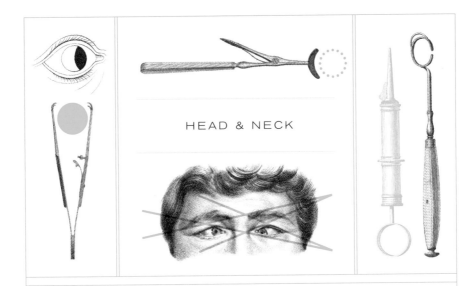

HEAD & NECK

II. *EYES.* 71

O. Muzzi.

Lit. Rudolf.

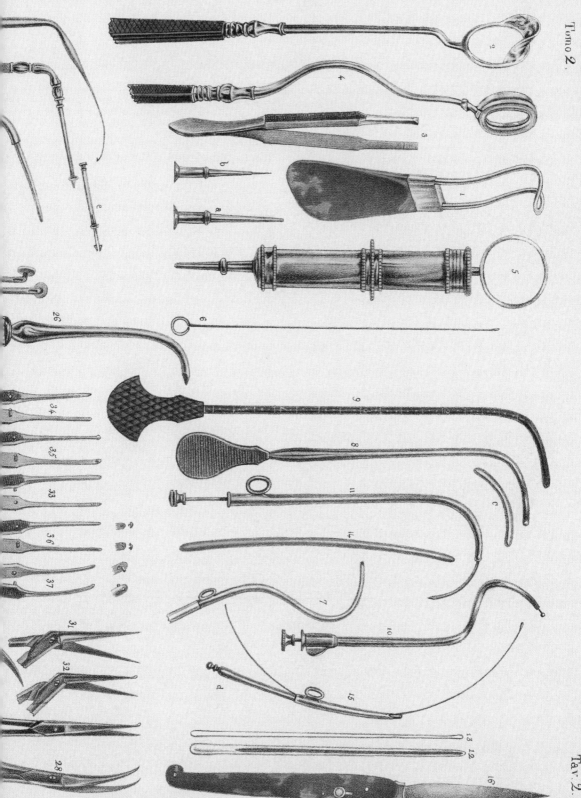

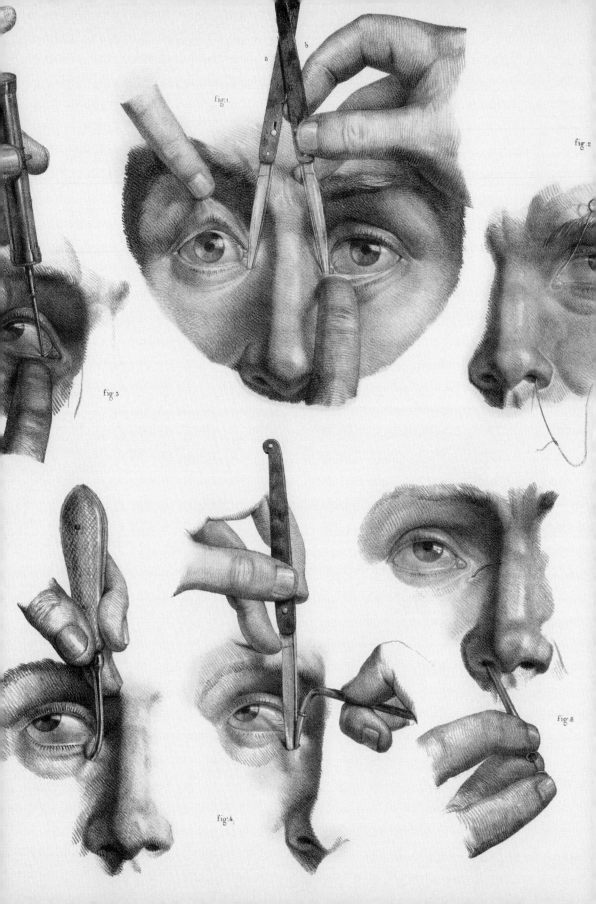

fig.1

fig.2

fig.3

fig.4

fig.6

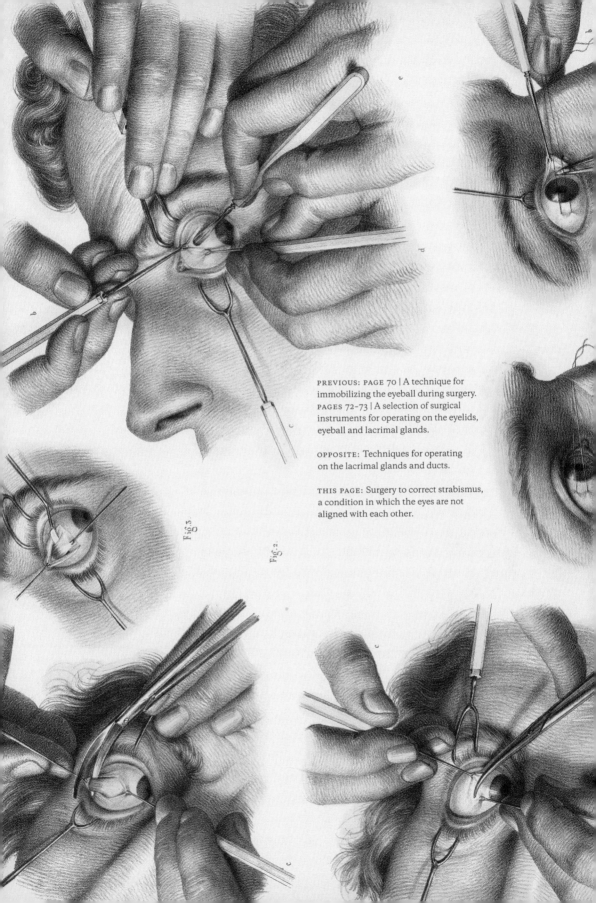

PREVIOUS: PAGE 70 | A technique for immobilizing the eyeball during surgery. PAGES 72-73 | A selection of surgical instruments for operating on the eyelids, eyeball and lacrimal glands.

OPPOSITE: Techniques for operating on the lacrimal glands and ducts.

THIS PAGE: Surgery to correct strabismus, a condition in which the eyes are not aligned with each other.

Fig.3.

Fig.2.

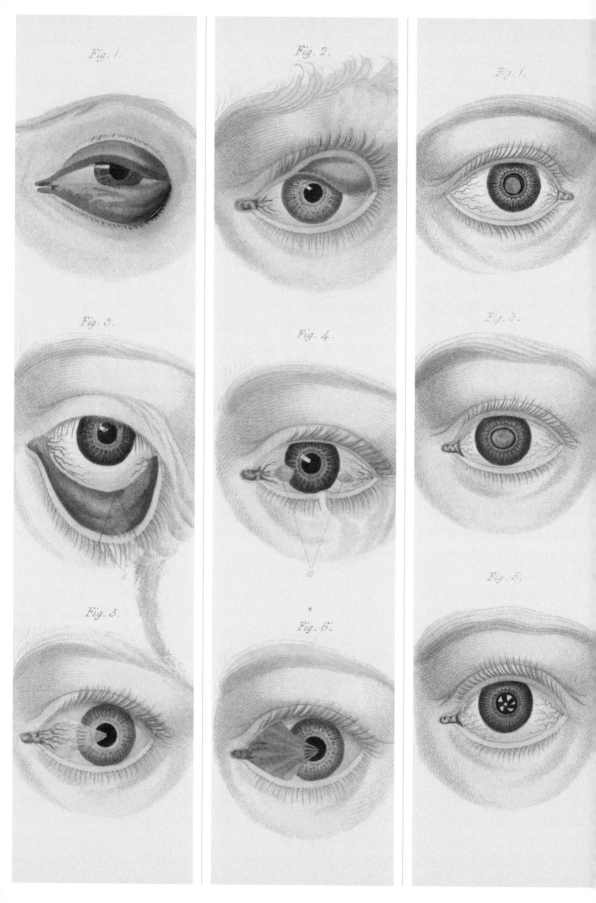

Fig. 1.

Fig. 2.

Fig. 1.

Fig. 3.

Fig. 4.

Fig. 3.

a

a

Fig. 5.

Fig. 6.

Fig. 5.

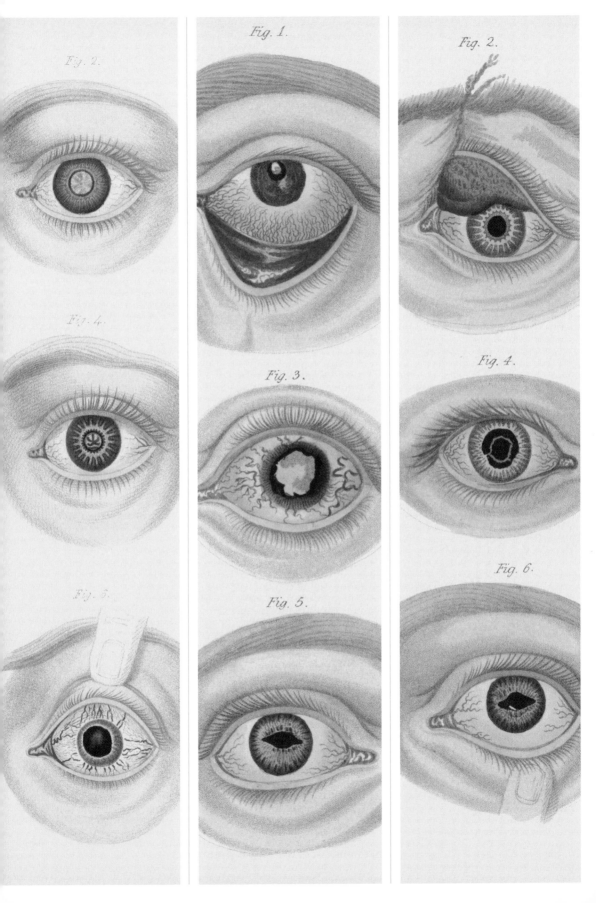

Fig. 2.

Fig. 1.

Fig. 2.

Fig. 4.

Fig. 3.

Fig. 4.

Fig. 6.

Fig. 5.

Fig. 6.

PREVIOUS: PAGE 76 (*left*) Two forms of eyelid eversion and a thin, membranous pterygium (benign growth of the conjunctiva). (*centre*) Two forms of eyelid eversion and a fleshy pterygium. (*right*) Two forms of cataract and a central opacity affecting the capsule of the eye.

PAGE 77 (*left*) Two forms of cataract and glaucoma. (*centre*) An eyelid inversion, cataract combined with glaucoma, and an artificial pupil created by excising a portion of the iris. (*right*) An eyelid inversion, a ring of opaque capsule, and an artificial pupil created by excising a portion of the iris.

THIS PAGE: Surgery on the lacrimal sac.

OPPOSITE: Surgery on the sclera of the eye and the extraocular muscles.

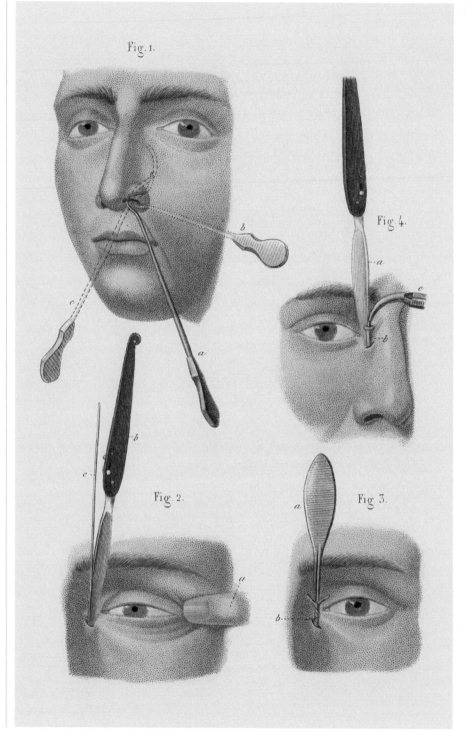

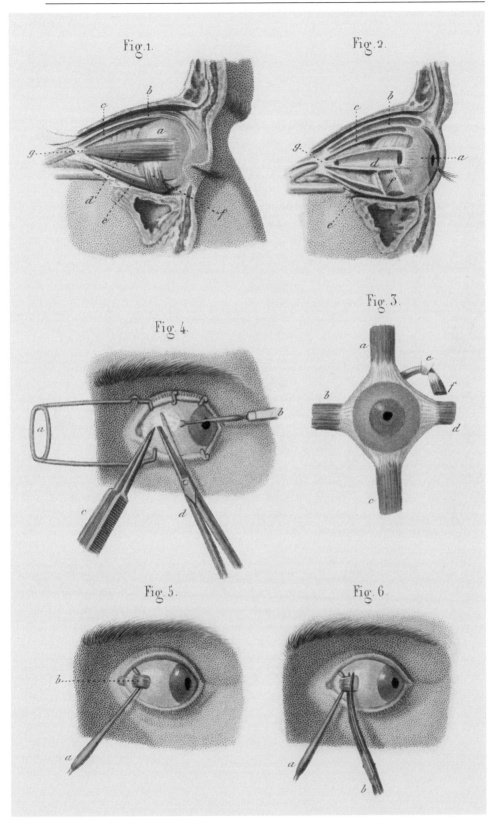

Fig. 1.

Fig. 2.

Fig. 3.

Fig. 4.

Fig. 5.

Fig. 6.

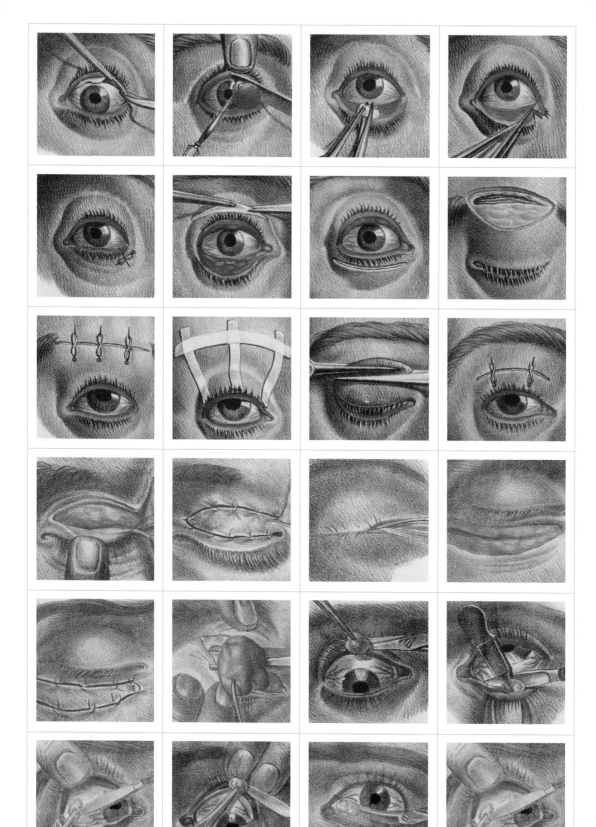

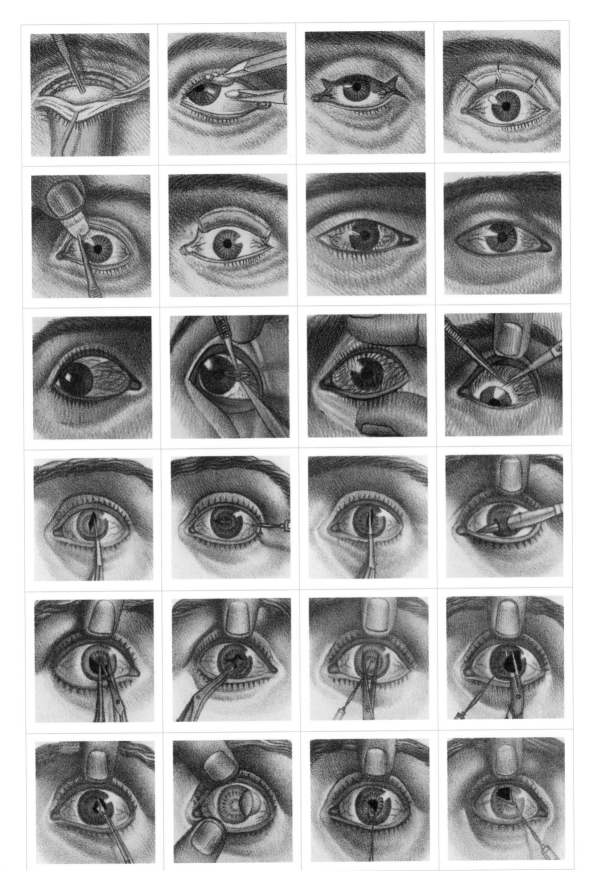

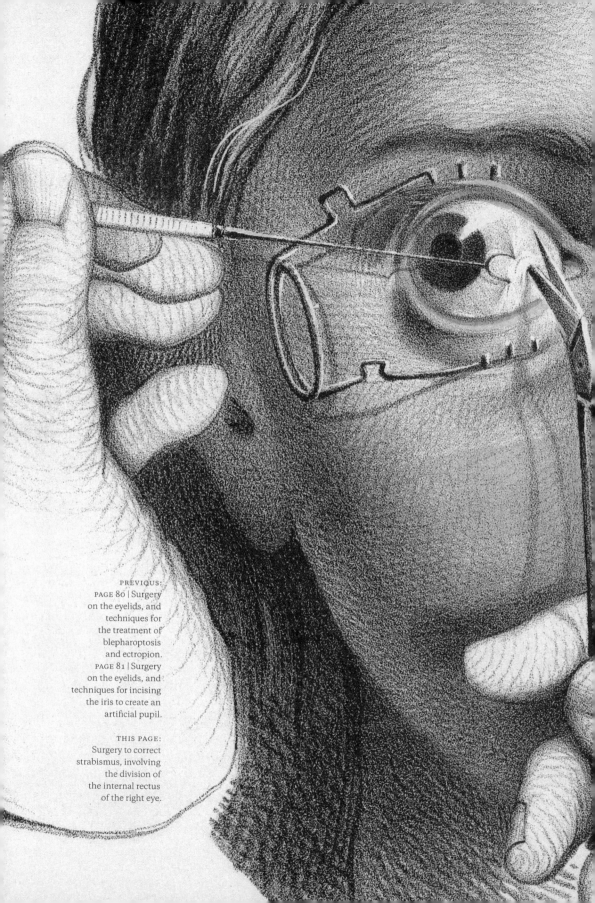

PREVIOUS:
PAGE 80 | Surgery
on the eyelids, and
techniques for
the treatment of
blepharoptosis
and ectropion.
PAGE 81 | Surgery
on the eyelids, and
techniques for
incising the iris to create an
artificial pupil.

THIS PAGE:
Surgery to correct
strabismus, involving
the division of
the internal rectus
of the right eye.

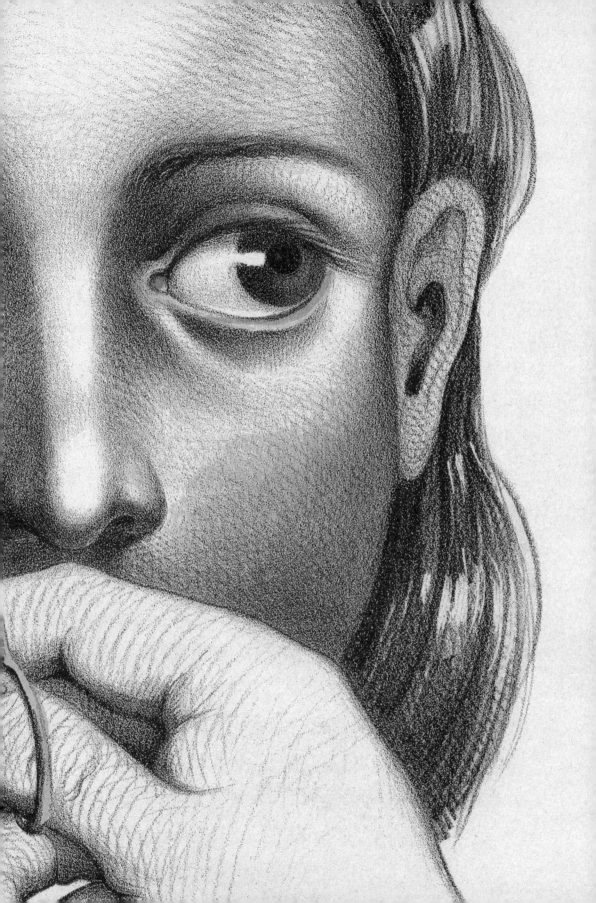

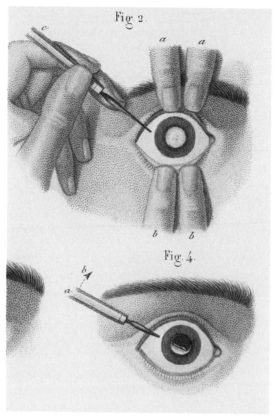

Fig. 2.

Fig. 4.

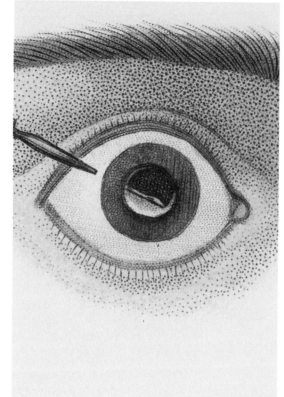

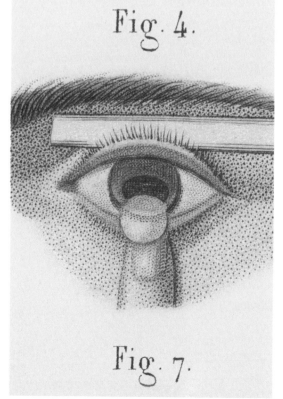

Fig. 4.

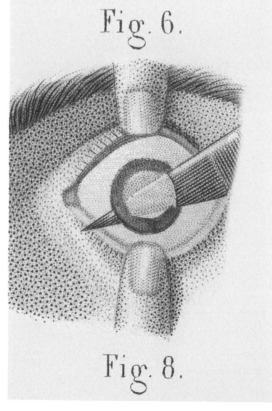

Fig. 6.

Fig. 7.

Fig. 8.

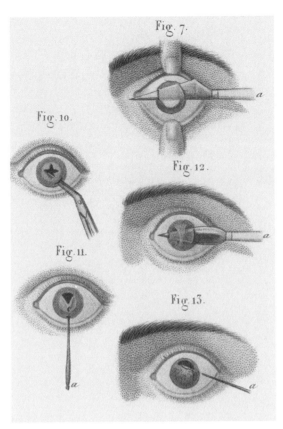

Fig. 7.

Fig. 10.

Fig. 12.

Fig. 11.

Fig. 13.

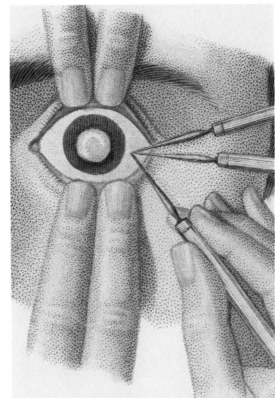

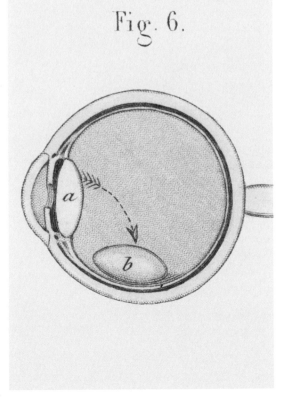

Fig. 6.

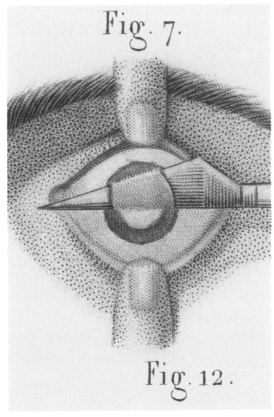

Fig. 7.

Fig. 12.

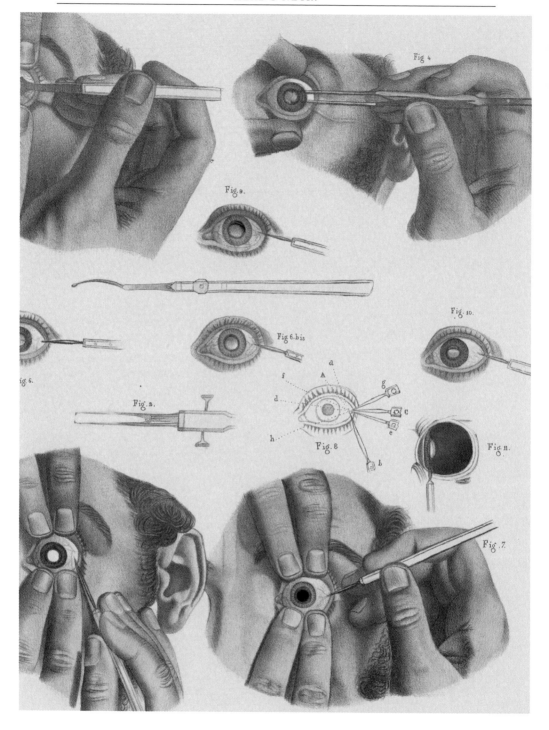

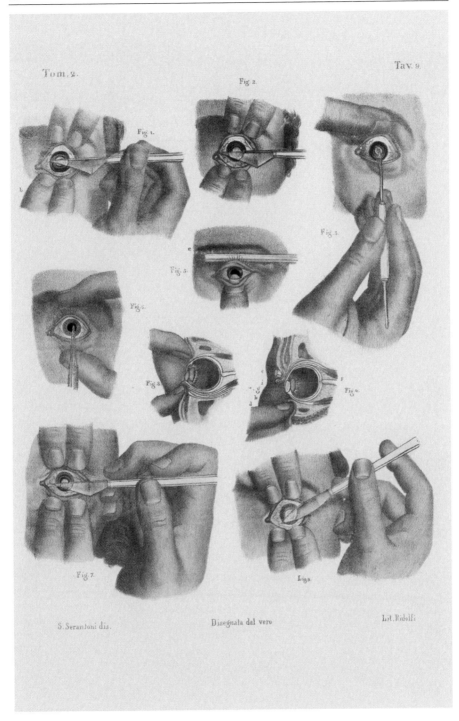

Tom. 2.   Fig. 2.   Tav. 9.

Fig. 1.

Fig. 3.

Fig. 5.

Fig. 6.

Fig. 3.

Fig. 4.

Fig. 7.   Fig. 8.

S. Serantoni dis.   Disegnata dal vero   Lit. Ridolfi

PREVIOUS, OPPOSITE & ABOVE: Techniques for the removal of cataracts.
OVERLEAF: Various techniques for operating on the upper and lower eyelids.

Fig. 1.

Fig. 2.

Fig. 3.

Fig. 4.

Fig. 5.

Fig. 6.

Fig. 7.

Fig. 8.

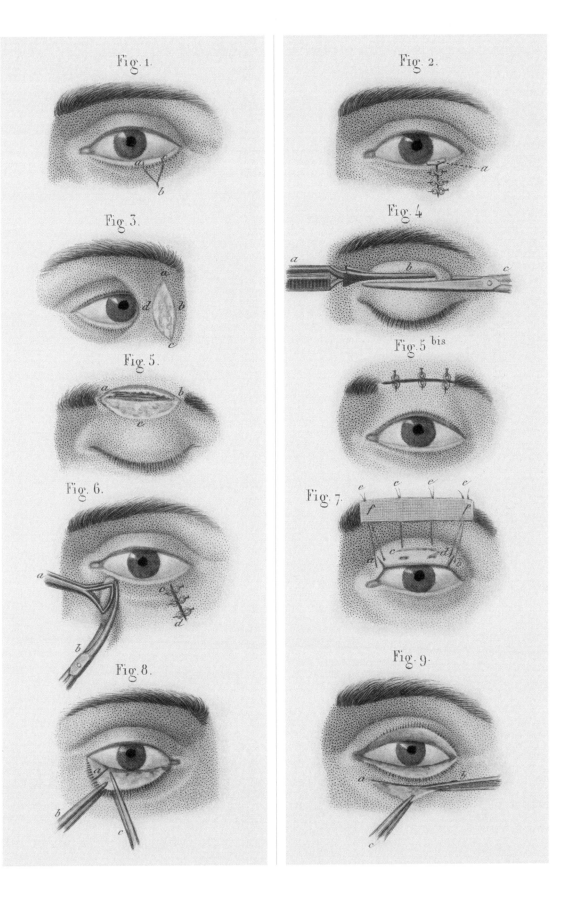

Fig. 1.

Fig. 2.

Fig. 3.

Fig. 4.

Fig. 5.

Fig. 5 bis

Fig. 6.

Fig. 7.

Fig. 8.

Fig. 9.

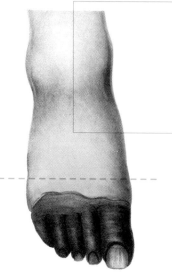

Fig. 1.

LET US SPRAY: *Antisepsis & the Hospital.*

Fig. 2.

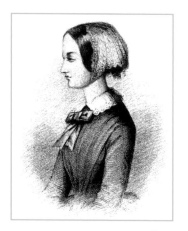

Fig. 3.

Even before the first general anaesthetics in 1847-67, surgeons in Europe and the United States were beginning to perform new operations in which they ventured into the abdomen and the chest. Those trained in the new Paris manner were keen to put their finely honed anatomo-localist knowledge to use, but no amount of operative skill seemed to reduce the risk of patients succumbing to gangrene or erysipelas. While anaesthesia made more invasive surgery acceptable to the public and the profession, antisepsis—a collection of techniques closely associated with the surgeon Joseph Lister—brought the notion of scientific surgery to public attention, and ultimately secured the status of hospitals as a bastion of surgical power.

By the middle of the nineteenth century, as politicians, physicians and civil engineers debated public health reform and the nature of infectious disease, some were beginning to ask whether industrial cities were really an appropriate place for hospitals. Influential voices such as James Young Simpson and Florence Nightingale—more on whom in *Ministers of Hygiene: Surgery & Nursing* (D; pages 142-147)—contrasted the 15 to 20 per cent mortality rate of amputations conducted in smaller provincial hospitals or in the homes of the wealthy with the 50 to 60 per cent mortality rate of the same procedure in large urban hospitals. In *Notes on Hospitals* (1859), Nightingale proposed that 'the very first requirement of a hospital is that it should do the sick no harm', and she and Simpson argued that city hospitals were themselves responsible for the sickness of their patients. Drawing on the Classical notion of infectious disease as a miasma—a poisonous emanation spreading from person to person through the air—they claimed that stagnant air in unventilated wards, along with miasmas from infected wounds and smoke from industrial chimneys, were poisoning hospital inmates. Simpson coined a term for this: 'hospitalism', defined by his colleague John Erichsen as 'a general morbid condition of the building, or its atmosphere, productive of disease'.

Nightingale's solution was to demolish dirty city hospitals and replace them with rural 'pavilion-hospitals', an idea originally put forward by the Parisian surgeon Jacques-René Tenon in the late eighteenth century. Tenon's pavilion-hospitals were single-storey wards with tall windows, connected by glazed corridors, and separated from one another by gardens. Good ventilation, regular fumigation, modern sewers, and—one factor that made his scheme particularly appealing to Nightingale—a strict routine for patients, nurses and physicians would eliminate hospitalism. Debates over the value of pavilion-hospitals crystallized around the rebuilding of St Thomas' Hospital in London in the 1860s. Nightingale's opponents pointed out the practical problems: could city-dwelling patients, doctors and surgeons really be expected to travel a dozen miles from home to give or receive treatment? A compromise saw St Thomas' rebuilt in the centre of London, with a view of the Palace of Westminster from across the Thames, but on a pavilion plan.

Many of Nightingale's opponents were surgeons, who saw her vision as a threat to their still insecure professional foothold in large urban teaching hospitals. The challenge facing Lister and his colleagues was not merely to solve the problem of post-operative wound infection, but to solve it in a way that validated both the idea of scientific surgery and the hospitals in which they had built their power base. Born in 1827 to a well-to-do Quaker family in Essex, Lister studied medicine at University College London and went on to hold a series of junior posts in Scottish teaching hospitals. In 1860,

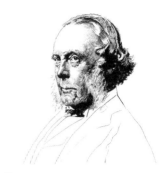

Fig. 4.

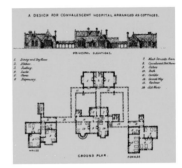

Fig. 5.

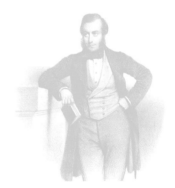

Fig. 6.

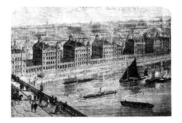

Fig. 7.

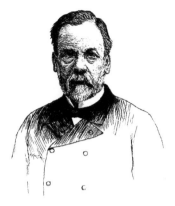

Fig. 8.

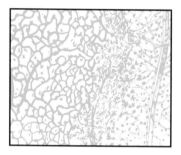

Fig. 9.

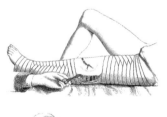

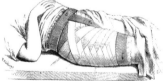

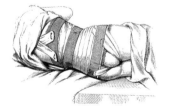

Fig. 10.

appointed regius professor of surgery at Glasgow, he encountered extremely high rates of surgical wound infection. His experiments on frogs showed that gangrene was related to environmental processes, like rotting. A paper by the French chemist Louis Pasteur, which argued that fermentation and food spoilage could be caused by microorganisms, led Lister to the idea that gangrene was caused by airborne bacteria entering wounds.

If this were the case, what could be done to keep wounds free from infection? Lister began to work with a substance already used in the processing of sewage— carbolic acid, a product of the new chemical industry, which experiments proved to be a potent antiseptic. On 12 August 1865, an eleven-year-old boy had been run over by a cart and brought into the Glasgow Royal Infirmary with a compound fracture of the tibia, the kind of injury most vulnerable to infection. Lister dressed the wound with lint soaked in a mixture of carbolic acid and linseed oil; six weeks later the boy walked out of the hospital, his leg completely healed. Over the next two years, Lister accumulated more cases, refined his procedure (using tinfoil to stop the dressing drying out), and in March 1867 published a description of his method in the *Lancet*.

Did this short article provoke an antiseptic revolution in Western surgery? No—and for several good reasons. Firstly, the notion of antisepsis had been in currency with physicians and surgeons for a long time, partly in the specific sense of dressing wounds with substances such as iodine in the hope of preventing suppuration, and partly in maintaining general cleanliness in hospitals to eliminate miasmas. Secondly, Lister did not intend his 1867 paper to be revolutionary, but merely a method for preventing infection in certain wounds. Finally—and most importantly—Lister's use of Pasteur's work was deeply controversial. Through the second half of the nineteenth century, physicians, surgeons and scientists continued to disagree over the nature of infectious disease, and even those who accepted that bacteria caused wound infections were not necessarily sympathetic to Pasteur's version of germ theory.

From 1860 the London surgeon T. S. Wells had been using what he called 'cleanliness and cold water' to fight wound infection. Wells claimed that by using fresh towels for each operation, rinsing his hands in cold water, and barring spectators who had attended an autopsy in the past week, he could achieve lower mortality rates than Lister. George William Callender, a surgeon at St Bartholomew's Hospital in the 1870s, reported an overall 3 per cent surgical mortality rate using 'cleanliness and cold water' compared with Lister's lowest figure of 15 per cent. This approach contrasted sharply with Lister's own distinction between 'aesthetic' and 'surgical' cleanliness, made in a speech in 1875:

> *It is now three years since any cleaning took place on these wards of mine… If we take cleanliness in any other sense than antiseptic cleanliness, my patients have the dirtiest wounds and sores in the world. I often keep on dressings for a week at a time, during which the discharge accumulates… Aesthetically they are dirty, though surgically clean.*

Over the following two decades, Lister gradually expanded his technique for dressing wounds into an entire surgical paradigm based on the antiseptic power of carbolic acid. He rinsed his hands and instruments in it before operating, and devised a steam-driven spray that would douse the operating field (along with the surgeon, his assistants and nurses) in carbolic acid while they operated. Listerian surgery seemed to work—his own mortality rates fell rapidly after 1865— and his model of surgery was taken up in France, Germany, Austria and Italy.

Surgeons who adopted Lister's method found it effective in reducing post-operative infection, but it produced an uncomfortable setting for surgery. The New York surgeon William Halsted was an enthusiastic proponent of antisepsis, but his colleagues hated the fumes from his carbolic spray and his operating theatre was exiled to a marquee in the garden of the Bellvue Hospital. Halsted's assistants developed 'carbolic coughs', and his chief nurse (and fiancée) Caroline

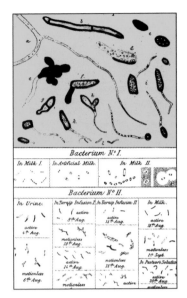

Fig. 11.

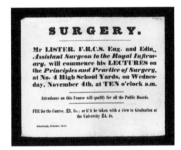

Fig. 12.

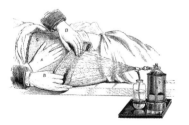

Fig. 13.

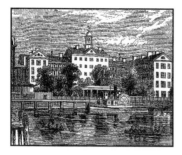

Fig. 14.

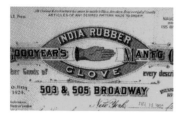

Fig. 15.

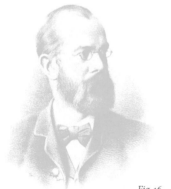

Fig. 16.

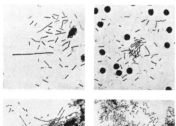

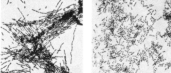

Fig. 17.

Hampton suffered painful dermatitis, relieved only when he persuaded the Goodyear Rubber Company to make her special gloves. Apart from its practical disadvantages, antisepsis also carried a more abstract risk. By focusing on the post-operative treatment of the wound, it made surgeons—rather than the hospital environment or the particular susceptibility of patients—responsible for infections.

The story of antisepsis also highlights the complexity of debates around germ theory and the influence of new views of disease on surgical practice. Seeking to reinforce the notion of scientific surgery, Lister constantly brought new ideas from laboratory science into his writings. His early view of infection drew heavily on Pasteur's work, but also on Classical ideas about wound healing: airborne germs entering the wound sparked the fermentation of dead tissue, interfering with the production of laudable pus, irritating exposed nerves and causing systemic fever. By 1881, Lister had abandoned this complex synthesis and the ancient idea of laudable pus, and endorsed the German bacteriologist Robert Koch's work on particular species of bacteria that entered wounds by physical contact.

By the end of the nineteenth century, Lister was feted around the world as the man who had made surgery safe and scientific, and as a living embodiment of Victorian ingenuity and rectitude. But his followers, while happy to work in what they called a Listerian tradition, treated his ideas pragmatically, adapting and even discarding his techniques. Robert Lawson Tait—a gifted surgeon who achieved low mortality rates, but also a committed opponent of germ theory—put it well in 1891:

> *The Listerism of twenty and fifteen and ten years ago is dead… We see the 'germicidians' coolly turn around and say 'our germicides were a joke; it was cleanliness we meant all the time.'*

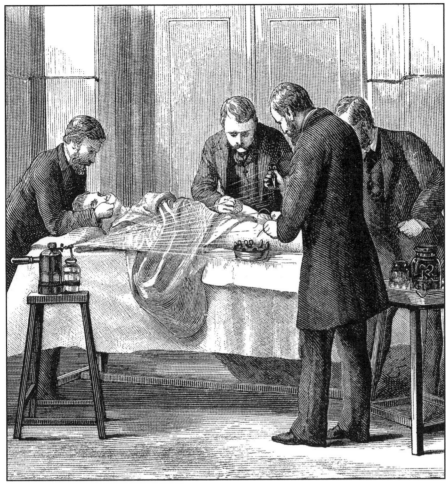

Fig. 18.

FIG. 1: *Gangrene and other 'hospital diseases' resulted in high post-operative death rates.* FIG. 2: *Florence Nightingale (1820-1910) came to embody Victorian ideals of cleanliness, godliness and order.* FIG. 3: *Nightingale's plan of the Scutari Hospital from 1855, at the beginning of her campaign to reform military nursing during the Crimean War (1853-1856).* FIG. 4: *Joseph Lister (1827-1912) as a Victorian 'Great Man', and the leader of British surgery.* FIG. 5: *Nightingale believed that efficiently run 'cottage' or 'pavilion hospitals' would eliminate the miasmas responsible for 'hospitalism'.* FIG. 6: *John Erichsen (1818-1896) argued that 'hospitalism' was a result of the dirty, polluted conditions in large urban hospitals.* FIG. 7: *The new St Thomas' Hospital, opened in 1868, used a pavilion plan, but in central London.* FIG. 8: *Lister's work on antisepsis initially drew on the ideas of French microbiologist Louis Pasteur (1822-1895).* FIG. 9: *Animal experiments—here on a frog's foot—helped to convince Lister that microorganisms cause wound inflammation and infection.* FIG. 10: *Antiseptic dressings, using lint soaked in carbolic acid, could be cumbersome.* FIG. 11: *Though Lister endorsed a germ theory of infection from the 1860s, his views changed radically over several decades.* FIG. 12: *Lister also drew on his practical experience as a surgeon in London, Glasgow and (here) Edinburgh.* FIG. 13: *In his early work, Lister relied on disinfectant carbolic acid—here, dressing a psoas abscess.* FIG. 14: *At Bellevue Hospital, New York, surgeons disagreed over the value of antiseptic surgery: effective but highly unpleasant.* FIG. 15: *Surgical rubber gloves made by the Goodyear Company mitigated the irritant effects of carbolic acid.* FIG. 16: *By the 1880s, the germ theory of German bacteriologist Robert Koch (1843-1910) was replacing Pasteur's version.* FIG. 17: *Koch's germ theory was based on specific strains of microorganisms, transmitted by physical contact rather than air.* FIG. 18: *Lister's steam-powered spray drenched the entire operating field in carbolic acid.*

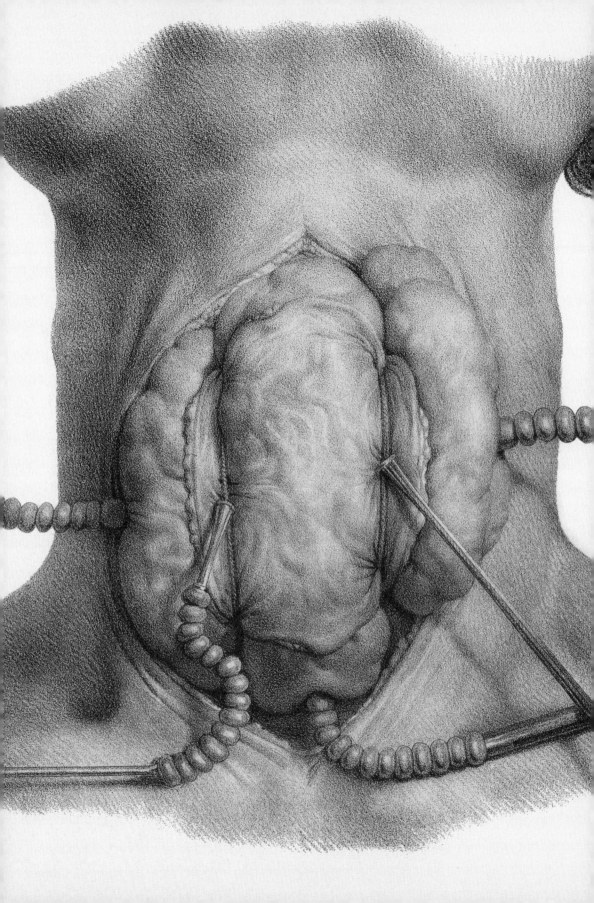

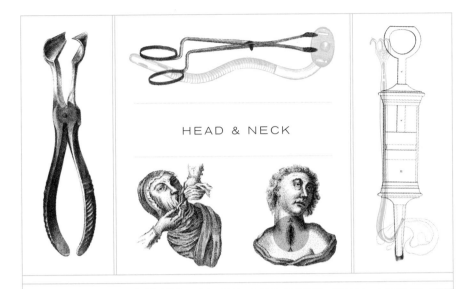

HEAD & NECK

EAR, NOSE & THROAT.

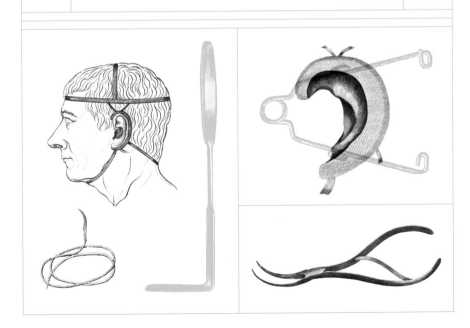

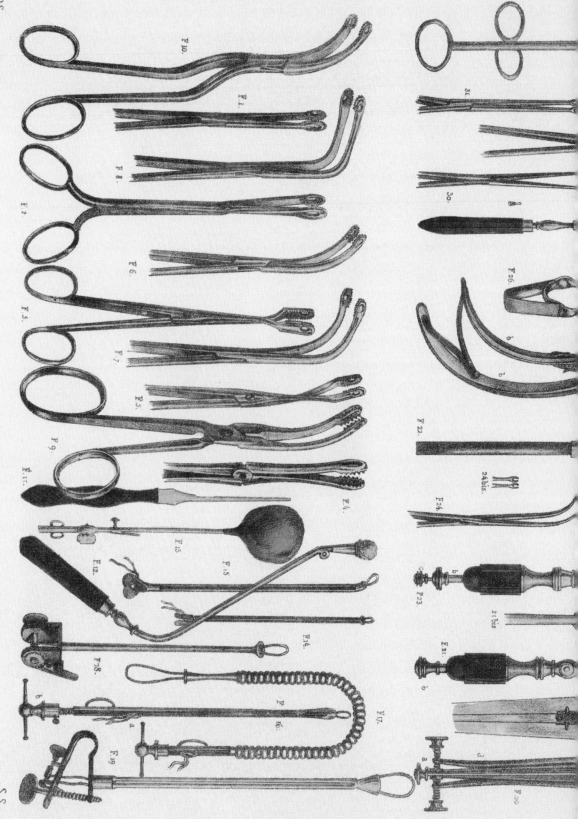

Lit. DS.

S. Scranton.

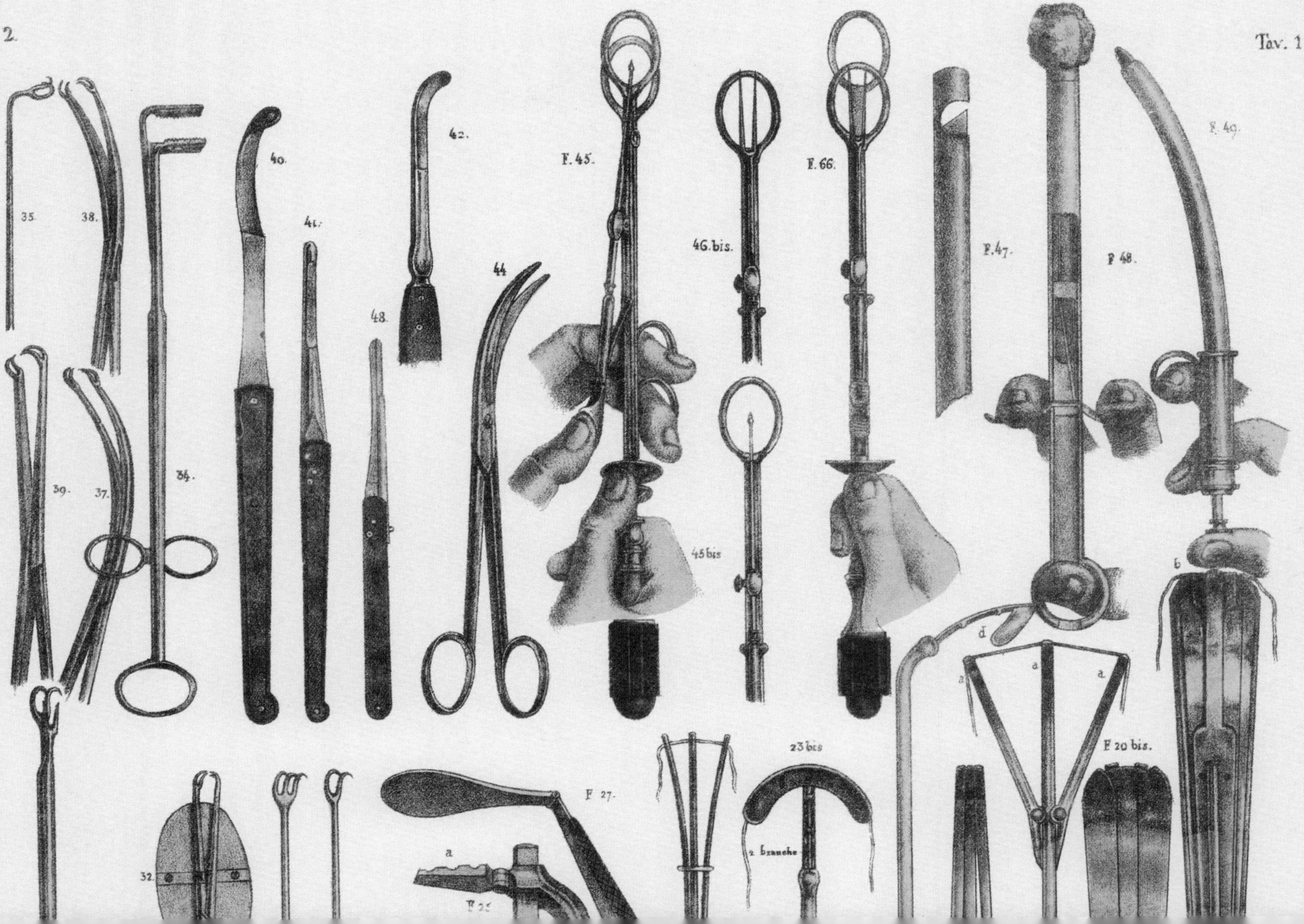
35.
38.
39.
37.
34.
40.
41.
48.
42.
44
F. 45.
45 bis
46.bis.
F. 66.
F. 47.
F 48.
F. 49.
b
d
a
a
a
F 20 bis.
23 bis
2 branche
F 27.
a
F 25
32.

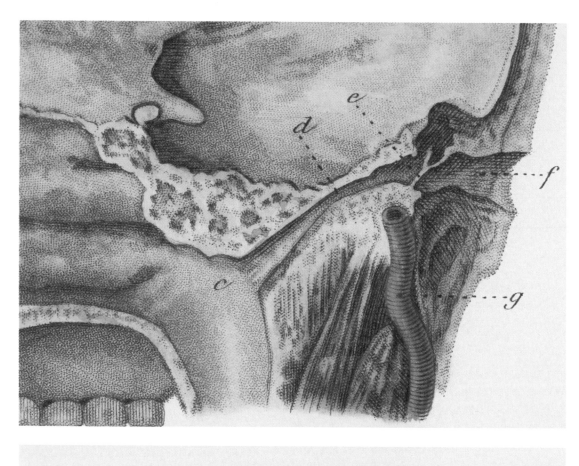

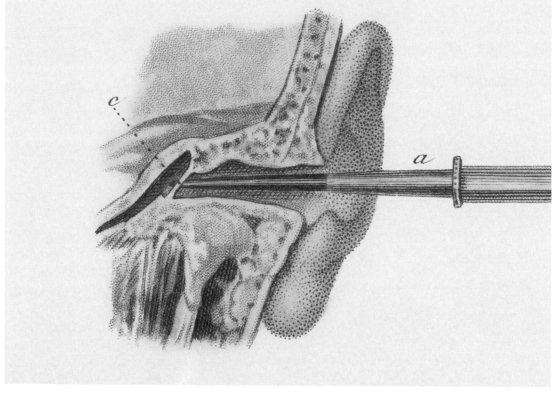

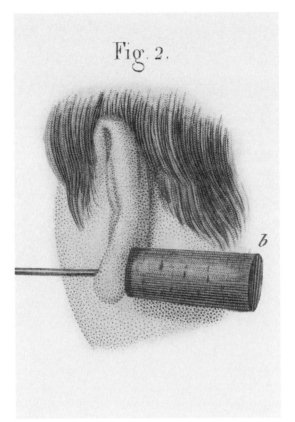

Fig. 2.

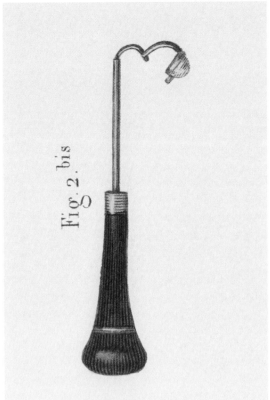

Fig. 2 bis

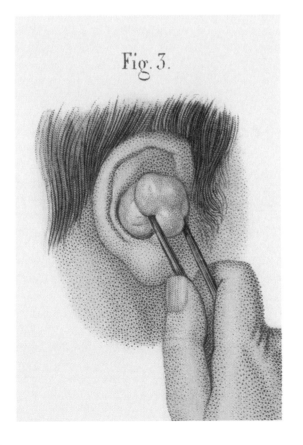

Fig. 3.

PREVIOUS: PAGE 96 | The removal
of a goitre (enlarged thyroid gland).
PAGES 98-99 | A selection of forceps,
clamps, scalpels and tonsil guillotines
used in throat surgery.

OPPOSITE: (*top*) The anatomy of the ear
canal and Eustachian tube. (*bottom*) An
instrument for operating on the eardrum.

THIS PAGE: (*top left*) A technique for
piercing the earlobe. (*top right*) An
instrument used in ear surgery. (*left*)
A tumour protruding from the right ear.

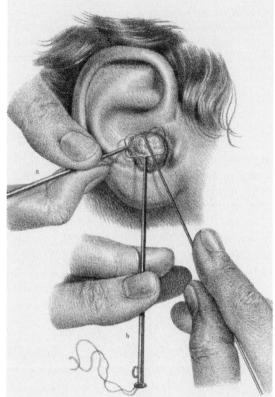

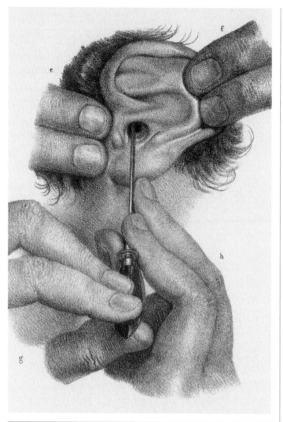

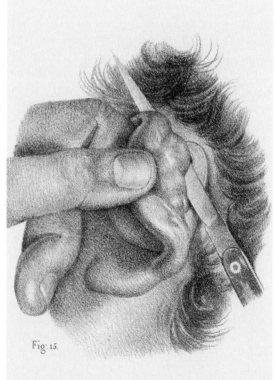

Fig. 15.

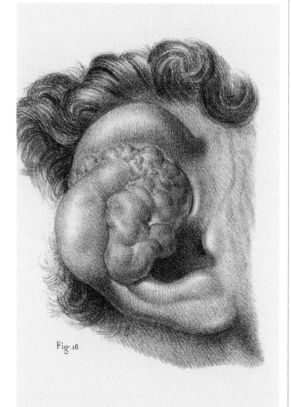

Fig. 16

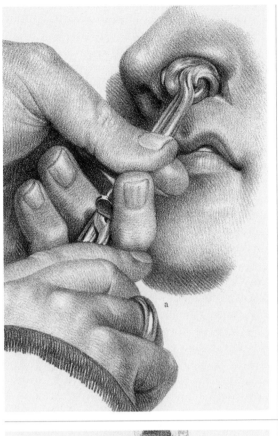

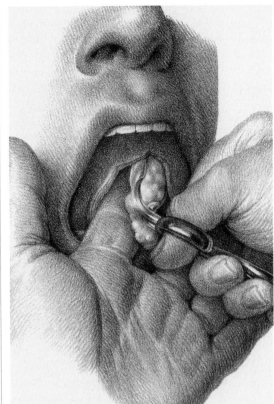

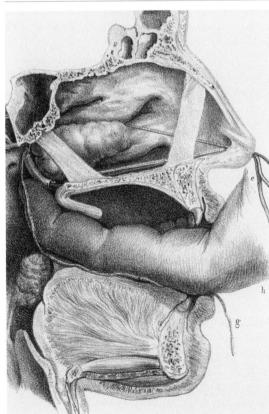

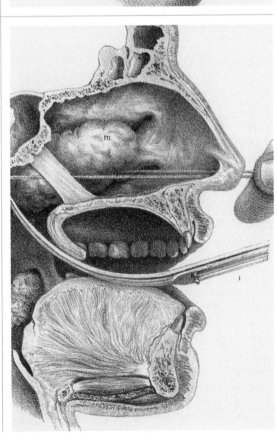

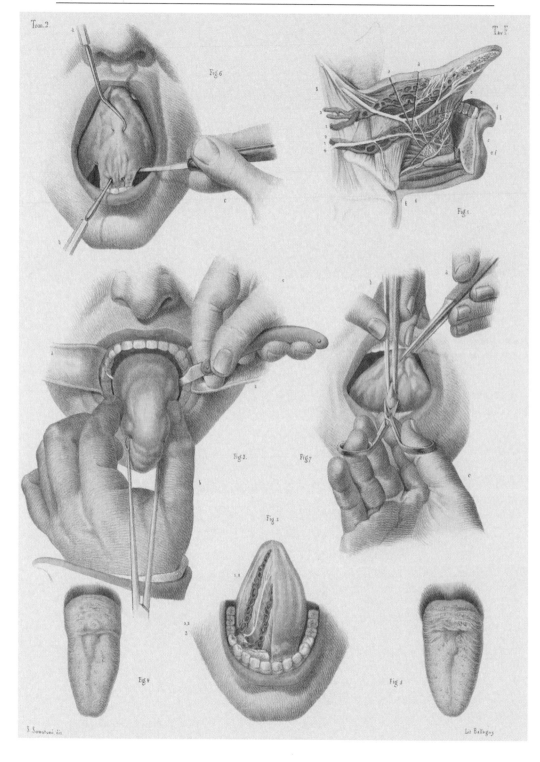

PREVIOUS: PAGE 102 | Instruments and techniques for operating on tumours of the ear. PAGE 103 | Instruments and techniques for operating on nasal polyps.

ABOVE & OPPOSITE: Anatomy of the tongue, and operative techniques and instruments used in surgery.

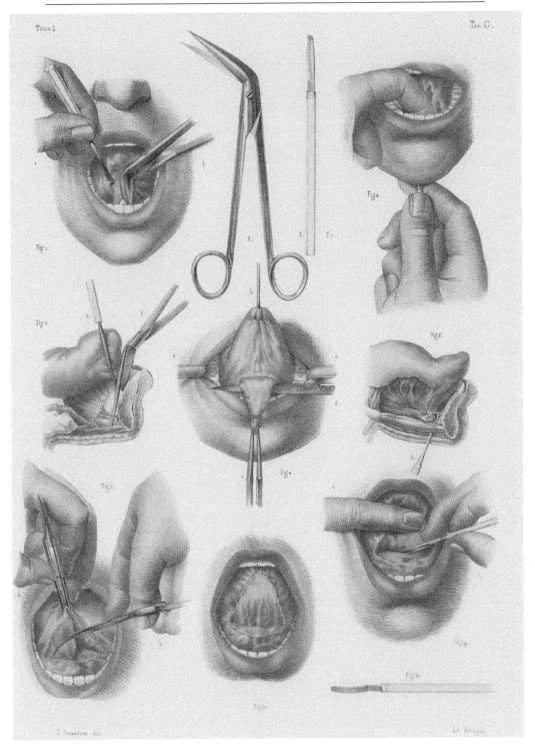

Tomo 2.

Tav. C.

Fig 1.

Fig 2.

Fig 3.

Fig 4.

Fig 5.

Fig 6.

Fig 7.

Fig 8.

Fig 9.

Fig 10.

Fig 11.

S. Serantoni dis.

Lit. Battaglini

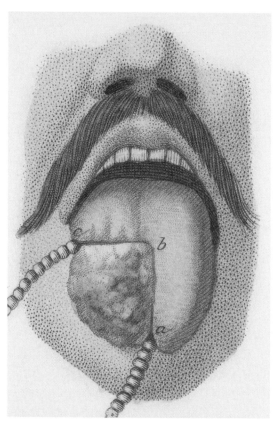

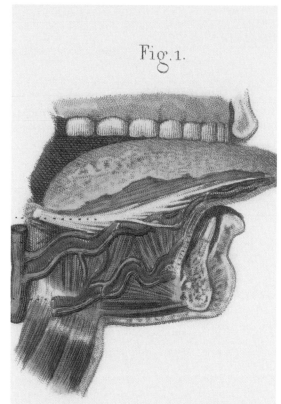

Fig.1.

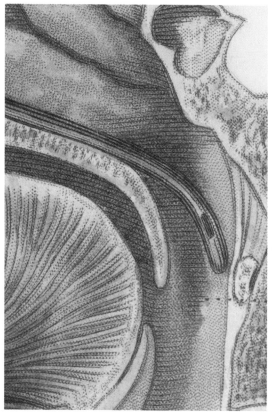

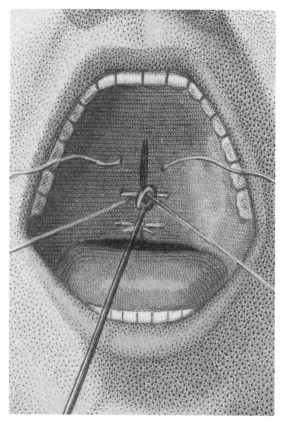

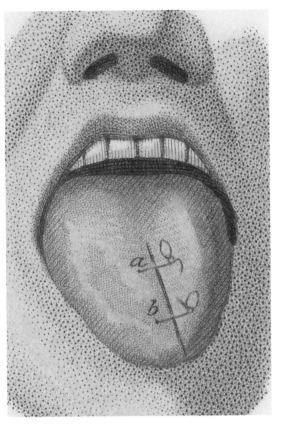

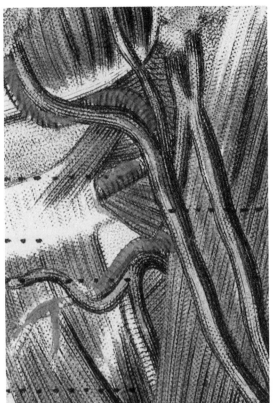

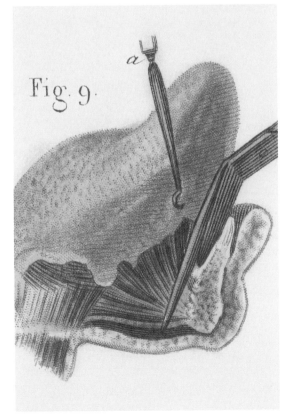

Fig. 9.

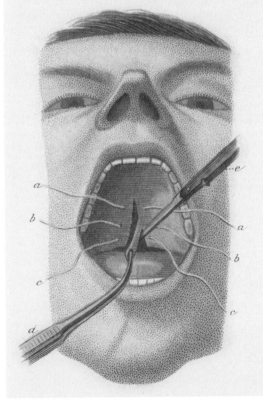

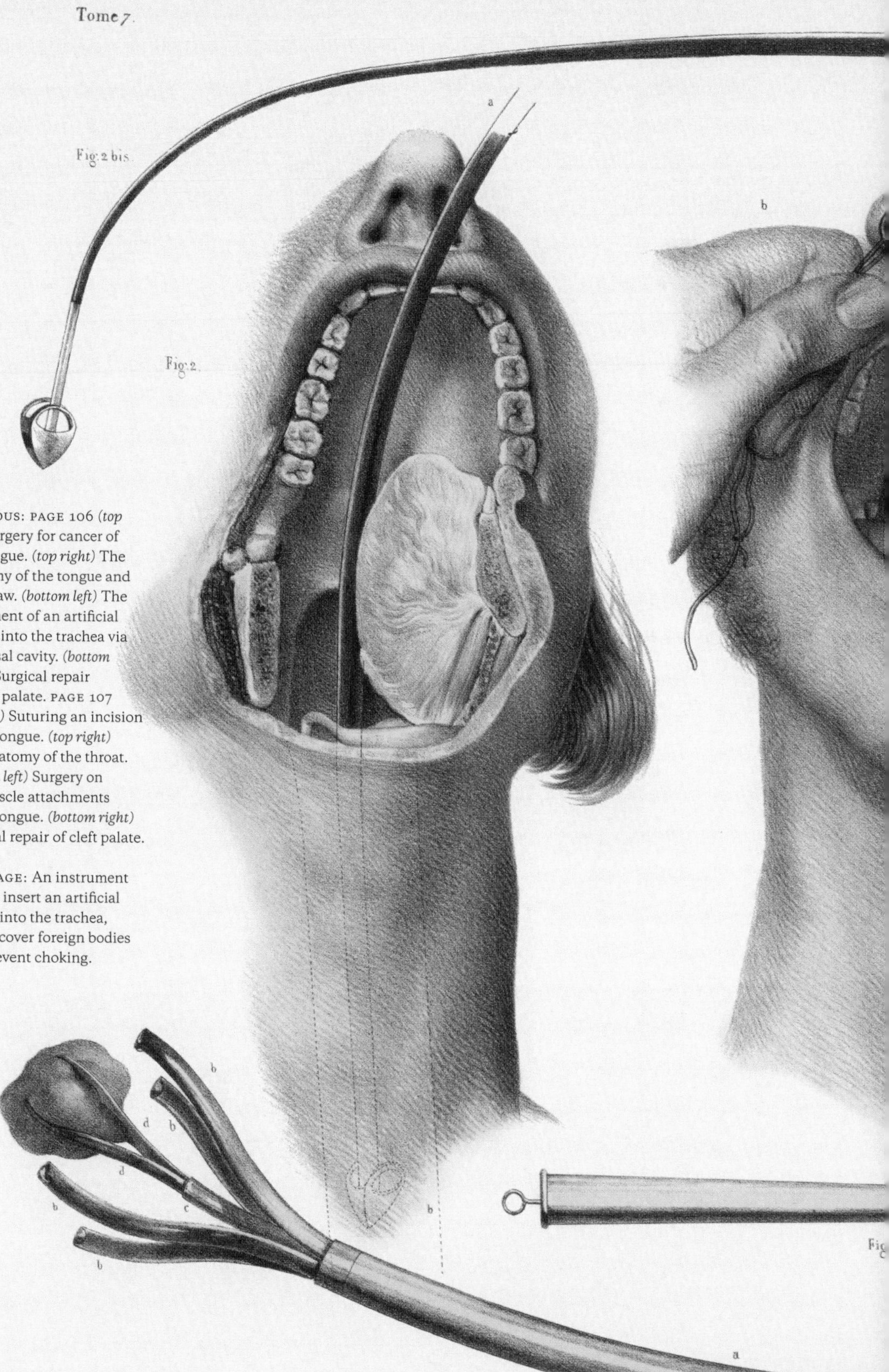

Fig. 2 bis.

Fig. 2.

PREVIOUS: PAGE 106 *(top left)* Surgery for cancer of the tongue. *(top right)* The anatomy of the tongue and lower jaw. *(bottom left)* The placement of an artificial airway into the trachea via the nasal cavity. *(bottom right)* Surgical repair of cleft palate. PAGE 107 *(top left)* Suturing an incision of the tongue. *(top right)* The anatomy of the throat. *(bottom left)* Surgery on the muscle attachments of the tongue. *(bottom right)* Surgical repair of cleft palate.

THIS PAGE: An instrument used to insert an artificial airway into the trachea, or to recover foreign bodies and prevent choking.

Bessme d'après nature par N.H.Jacob.

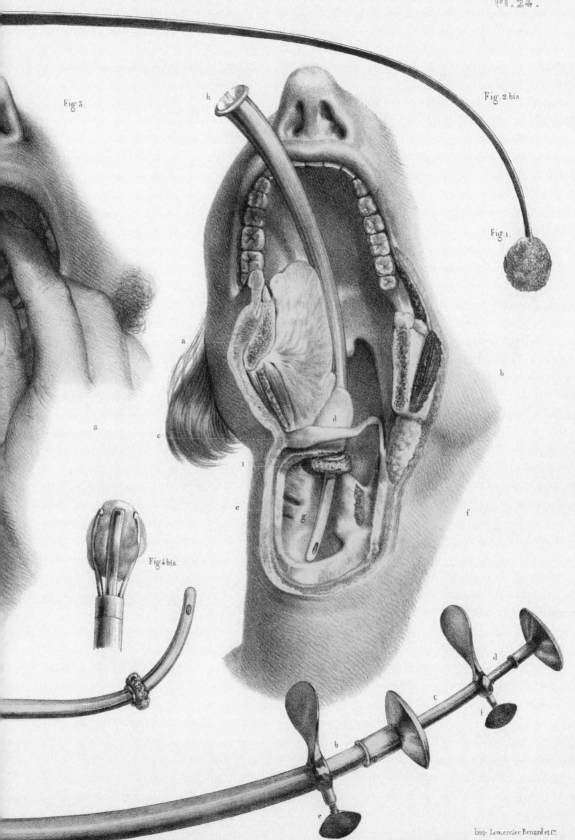

Pl. 24.

Fig. 3.

Fig. 2 bis.

Fig. 1.

a

b

a

c

d

i

e

g

f

h

Fig. 4 bis.

d

c

f

b

e

Imp. Lemercier-Benard et Cie.

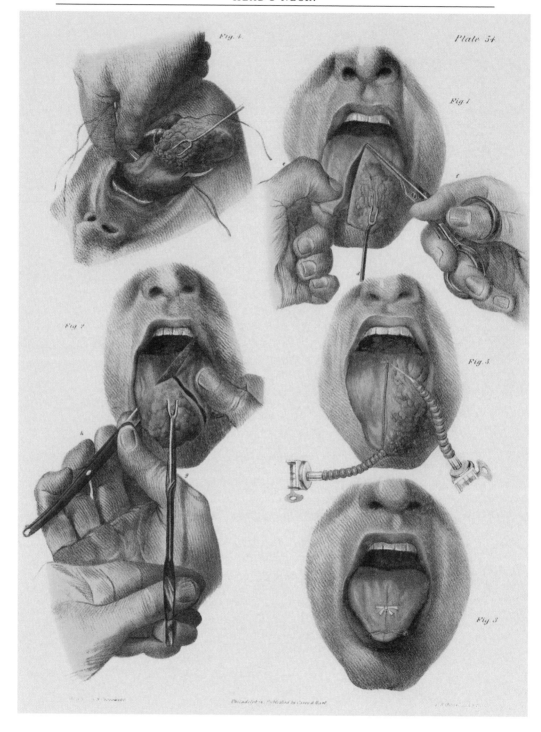

ABOVE: Surgery for cancer of the tongue.
OPPOSITE: Surgery for cleft palate, and tracheotomy.

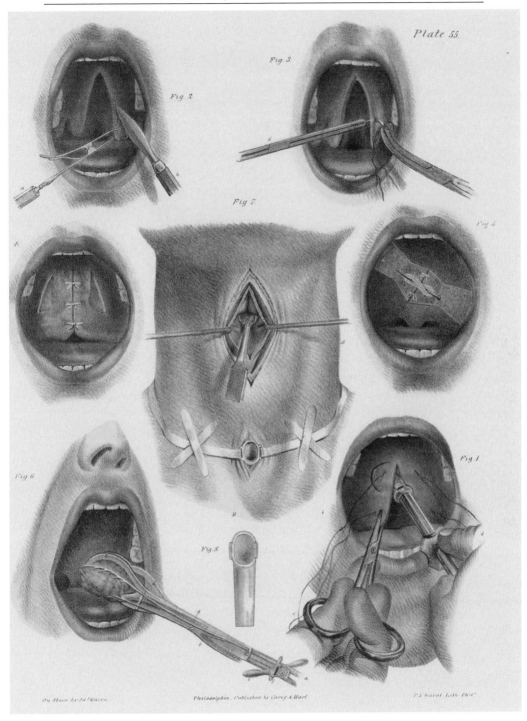

Plate 10.

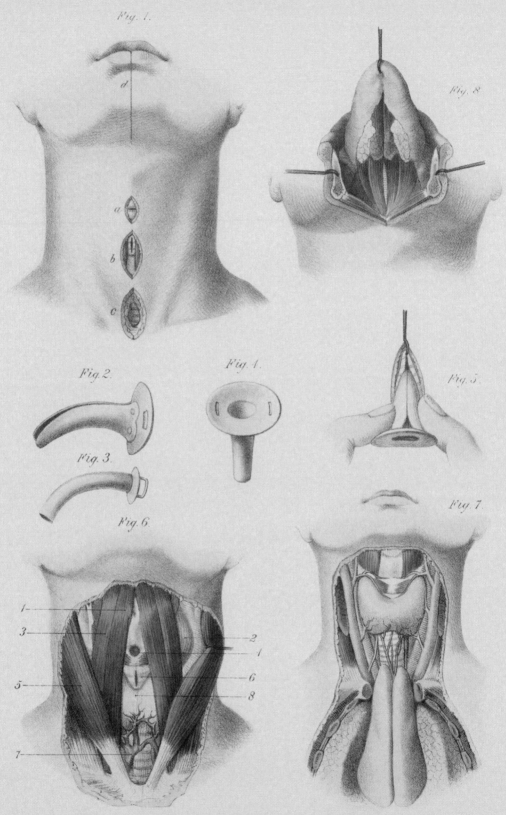

Fig. 1.

d

a

b

c

Fig. 8.

Fig. 2.

Fig. 3.

Fig. 4.

Fig. 5.

Fig. 6.

Fig. 7.

1

3

5

7

2

4

6

8

C Heath præp.   J.B. Leveillé del ad nat. 1875.   Hanhart lith

Plate 5.

OPPOSITE: Anatomy of the lower jaw and neck, and tracheotomy with insertion of artificial airways.

THIS PAGE: Anatomy of the neck, and ligature of arteries.

OVERLEAF: PAGE 114 (*top left*) A view of the mouth, tongue and tonsils. (*top centre*) Ligature technique for the removal of a goitre. (*top right*) Anatomy of the tongue. (*centre left*) Anatomy of the neck, showing locations for an incision in the oesophagus. (*centre*) Locations for ligating the common carotid, lingual and facial arteries. (*centre right*) Technique for removing swollen tonsils. (*bottom left*) Technique for removing nasal polyps. (*bottom centre*) Ligature technique for the removal of a goitre. (*bottom right*) Repair of a fistula in the parotid duct. PAGE 115 (*top left*) Anatomy of the neck, showing locations for a tracheotomy. (*top centre*) Anatomy of the mouth and pharynx, for surgery on the lacrimal sac. (*top right*) The removal of a tumour by passing a needle and suture through its base. (*centre left*) Technique for making an incision in the oesophagus. (*centre*) Anatomy of the major arteries and veins around the trachea, for tracheotomy. (*centre right*) Surgical removal of a tumour on the tongue. (*bottom left*) A tracheotomy and artificial airway held in place with sticking plaster. (*bottom centre*) The anatomy of the tongue and lower jaw. (*bottom right*) Anatomy of the neck and thyroid gland, for tracheotomy.

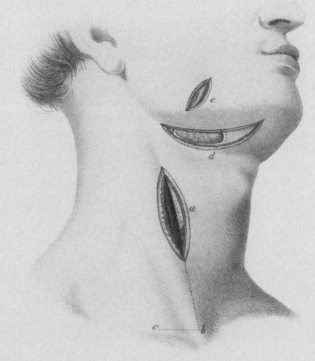

Fig. 1.

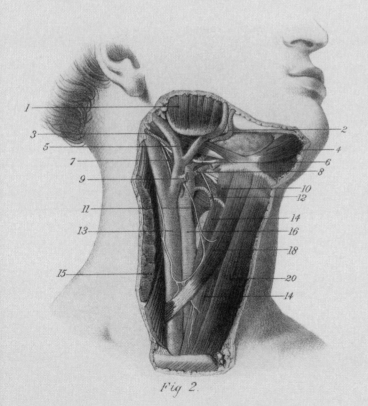

Fig 2.

C.Heath præp J.B.Léveillé del ad nat. 1875. Hanhart lith.

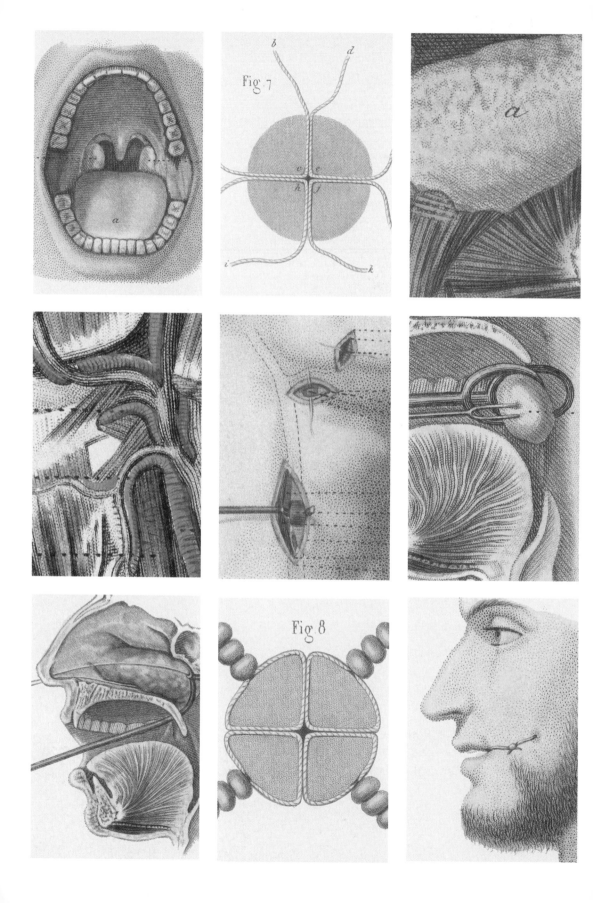

Fig. 7

Fig 8

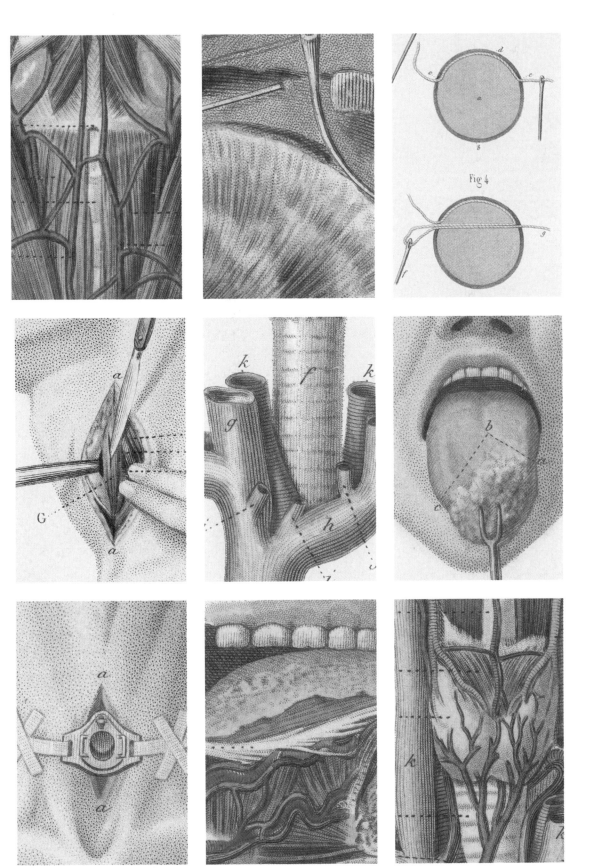

Fig 4

SCRUBBING UP: *Asepsis & the Operating Theatre.*

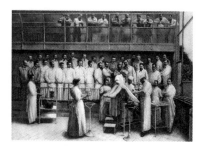

Fig. 1.

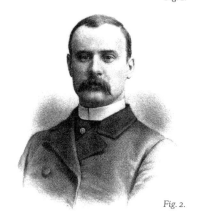

Fig. 2.

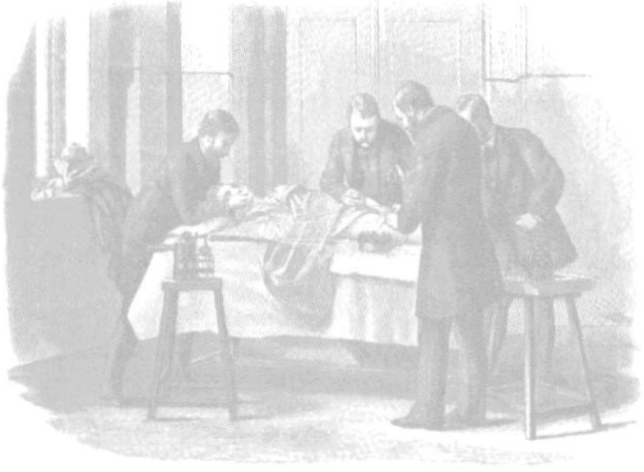

Fig. 3.

In a lecture on 'The Surgery of the Peritoneum', delivered in October 1896, the surgeon Frederick Treves ridiculed the latest fashion in French and German surgery:

> *In this practical country we have fortunately been spared the extravagances which have brought certain Continental operating theatres into ridicule. Those who come after us will read with interest of the operating theatre built like a diving tank, of the glass table for the patient, of the exquisite ceremony of washing on the part of the operator, of the rites attending the ostentatious cleansing of the patient, of the surgeon in his robes of white mackintosh and his india-rubber fishing boots, and of the onlookers beyond the pale who are excluded with infinite solicitude, from the sacred circle as septic outlaws. This exhibition may be scientific, but it is no part of surgery.*

Mid nineteenth-century public health reformers had sought to tackle urban poverty and sickness by cleaning up the industrial cities. Late nineteenth-century surgeons applied the same rationale—with a very different theoretical basis—to the spaces in which they worked.

Joseph Lister's antisepsis had been concerned with killing bacteria in surgical wounds, and as such did not demand a special operating environment. Antiseptic surgery could be carried

out in the homes of patients (as long as they did
not object to their carpets and furniture getting
a drenching with carbolic acid) or in large old-
fashioned operating theatres, and surgeons
continued to operate in their street clothes. By
contrast, the goal of aseptic surgery was to exclude
microorganisms from the surgical environment,
and its sphere of influence moved out from the
operating field to the bodies of surgeons and
assistants, their clothing and equipment, and
eventually to the operating theatre itself. Under
the regime of asepsis, operating theatres—like
nineteenth-century laboratories—became sites of
standardization and control, a setting in which the
ideal conditions for safe scientific surgery could be
established and maintained. And this did not end
at the doors of the theatre. From now on, hospital
laundries and autoclaves, nurses, architects, soap
suppliers and even the putty in window frames were
a bacteriological front line, each responsible for the
protection of patients.

The intellectual origins of aseptic practice lay
in a shift in European bacteriological thinking,
from the work of the French chemist Louis
Pasteur—for whom infections were spread by non-
specific airborne bacteria—to that of the German
physician Robert Koch, who identified specific
strains of skin-dwelling microorganisms as the
cause of most wound infections. Pasteur was first to
propose that surgeons adopt the rigorous practices
of sterilization and cleanliness in laboratories, in an
1878 essay on 'The Germ Theory and its Application
to Medicine and Surgery'. For the first generation
of aseptic surgeons, however, Koch's 'Studies on
the Aetiology of Wound Infection', published in the
same year, provided the compelling rationale for
aseptic practice.

Koch's work also cast doubt on the practical
value of antiseptic surgery. In 1881 he showed that
the dilutions of carbolic acid commonly used by
Listerian surgeons would take days, rather than
minutes, to kill bacterial spores, and so were useless

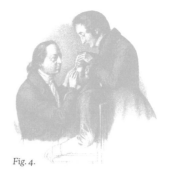

Fig. 4.

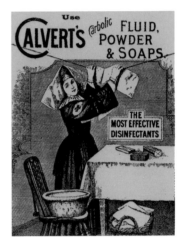

Fig. 5.

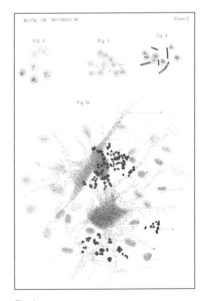

Fig. 6.

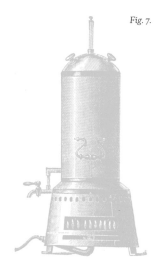

Fig. 7.

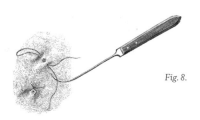

Fig. 8.

[1] Thomas Schlich, 'Surgery, science and laboratories as spaces of control', *History of Science 45*, 2007, 231-256.

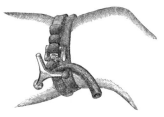

Fig. 9.

for sterilizing tools or hands. As an alternative he suggested corrosive sublimate, and Lister dutifully adopted it in his practice, but even this had its problems: it attacked steel tools, and if used over-generously could leave patients with mercury poisoning. Koch's favoured approach, set out in another 1881 paper, was to sterilize instruments and dressings with boiling steam.

Unlike antisepsis, asepsis was never identified with a single founding practitioner. A diverse set of aseptic techniques emerged gradually throughout the 1880s and 1890s, as surgeons across Europe began to engage with Koch's ideas. From 1886 surgeons at the Ziegelstrasse Klinik in Berlin were using autoclaved dressings and instruments, and a few years later the Swiss surgeon Emil Theodor Kocher began to suture wounds with sterilized silk thread. Their methods reached a wider audience through the tenth International Medical Congress, held in Berlin in 1890, and a year later the physician Curt Schimmelbusch published a *Guide to the Aseptic Treatment of Wounds*, which drew these techniques together under the label of asepsis. In the year of the congress, Lister himself abandoned the carbolic spray and acquired an autoclave, and his English colleague Berkeley Moynihan adopted a rigorous ritual of 'scrubbing up' before operations.

Surgeons' growing endorsement of germ theory, though, does not entirely explain the appeal of aseptic practice. Thomas Schlich has argued that the ideology of control became central to late nineteenth-century scientific surgery: infection control through antisepsis or asepsis; control of haemorrhage through new forceps, ligatures and tourniquets; and control of the patient through anaesthesia.[1] Just as laboratory scientists aimed to regulate experimental variables, so surgeons sought to manage and manipulate the bodies of their patients, and (vice versa) experimental physiologists borrowed surgical techniques. Anaesthesia and antisepsis not only reduced suffering in animal vivisection studies, but also

minimized stress and disturbance, allowing
researchers to collect more accurate data on the
functioning of organs during experiments. And just
as laboratory scientists worked under a physically
and intellectually demanding regime, so asepsis
placed intense new pressures upon surgeons.
Asepsis called for the absence of germs, not the
presence of carbolic acid, and any contamination
of the surgical environment, no matter how trifling,
might lead to infection. Surgical success now
relied on trust in the people and machines given
responsibility for sterilization.

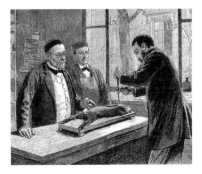

Fig. 10.

One outcome of this new concern with control
was the look of the modern operating theatre. Until
the late nineteenth century, operating theatres
were well-named: tiered ranks of seats rose around
a wooden bench, marking out a space in which a
crowd of spectators witnessed dramatic triumphs
and tragedies. Under the influence of asepsis, these
old theatres disappeared. Spectators represented a
potent source of infection, and saw-bitten wooden
benches could hardly be sterilized to laboratory
standards. New theatres were cleaner and quieter;
controlled spaces to which only those involved in
operations had access. Walls were tiled; corners
were rounded out so that dirt would not accumulate;
patients lay on steel or glass tables; ventilation and
temperature were regulated by some of the first air-
conditioning units; and electric lamps saturated the
operating field in light. Even the location of theatres
within hospitals began to change: aseptic surgeons
preferred top-floor rooms, away from the dirt and
noise of the street.

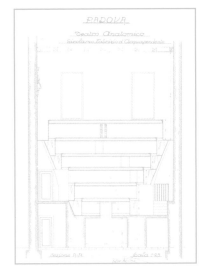

Fig. 11.

Under this exacting regime, new surgical
instruments, too, were reinvented. Surviving Greek
and Roman tools show that the basic forms of
operative kit had changed little over two thousand
years. Had he stepped into a mid eighteenth-
century operating theatre, Galen might have
recognized most of the knives and probes, saws
and forceps in use. By the end of the eighteenth
century, as the status of surgery rose, specialist

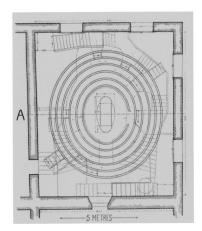

Fig. 12.

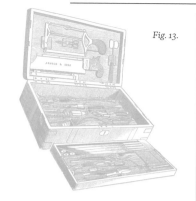

Fig. 13.

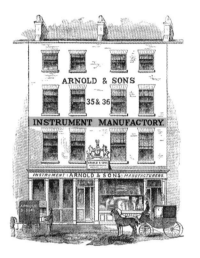

Fig. 14.

[2] Christopher Lawrence, 1992.

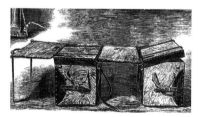

Fig. 15.

instrument-makers began to appear in the larger cities. Experienced hospital practitioners might commission special tools to suit their hands or their clientele; surgeon-apothecaries or naval surgeons might invest in the classic surgical set of a saw, knives and a trepanation drill, cased like duelling pistols in a velvet-lined teak box. Bloodily effective they may have been, but these ornate wooden-handled tools went the way of the public operating theatre. By the 1890s, surgeons favoured clean-lined scalpels and probes forged in stainless steel. Some practical-minded surgeons preferred to fabricate their own tools and, as late as 1915, surgical textbooks included instructions for tempering, brazing and soldering.

Along with new operating theatres and new tools came, gradually, a lightness of touch. Surgeons found that wounds made gently and carefully healed with less scarring, and methodical clamping of vessels could greatly reduce blood loss. In this way, asepsis went along with another shift in surgical identity: surgeons were coming to see themselves as meticulous scientists, rather than courageous fighters, working in a hushed and spotless surgical laboratory. Through the rigours of aseptic control and the rituals of scrubbing up, surgeons 'began to perceive themselves as "apart from and above" their colleagues'.[2]

At the beginning of the twentieth century, not all Western surgeons practised asepsis. Large teaching hospitals had adopted the idea, and taught it to their students, but how could these exacting techniques be adapted for use on battlefields or colonial frontiers? Even in less demanding settings, such as the general surgery practised well into the twentieth century by country GPs, old-fashioned chloroform and antisepsis continued to save the lives of many patients.

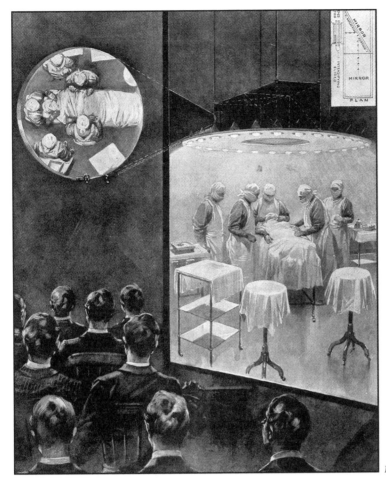

Fig. 16.

FIG. 1: *This 1901 print shows that even after aseptic surgery had been widely adopted, operating theatres could still be crowded places.* FIG. 2: *Frederick Treves (1853–1923), surgeon to King Edward VII and opponent of what he saw as the excesses of aseptic surgery.* FIG. 3: *Lister's antiseptic surgery did not require a special operating environment: this 1882 print shows surgeons operating in the patient's house.* FIG. 4: *The rise of asepsis ended the centuries-old practice of surgeons operating in their day clothes, as in this 1843 illustration of cataract removal.* FIG. 5: *Soap manufacturers were quick to capitalize on Lister's antiseptic surgery: this 1888 advert claims carbolic soap as 'the most effective disinfectant'.* FIG. 6: *Koch's bacteriological studies showed that carbolic acid was comparatively ineffective at killing the germs responsible for septicaemia and wound infections.* FIG. 7: *Instead of chemical disinfectants, Koch recommended the sterilization of instruments and dressings with boiling steam.* FIG. 8: *Sutures such as these could be a dangerous source of infection if they were inadequately sterilized or wrongly inserted.* FIG. 9: *The discipline of asepsis also encouraged a gentler approach to surgery, and the abandonment of effective but damaging instruments such as this tourniquet.* FIG. 10: *Pasteur's germ theory formed the basis of his practical work on vaccines for diseases such as rabies (demonstrated here).* FIG. 11: *For centuries, operating and anatomy theatres were literally theatres, with tiers of seats surrounding a stage.* FIG. 12: *In the famous anatomy theatre at Padua, all spectators could get a good view.* FIG. 13: *Cased surgical kits such as these were effective operative tools, but proved extremely difficult to sterilize with carbolic acid or steam.* FIG. 14: *In the late nineteenth century, instrument-makers such as Arnold & Sons of London began to design new surgical tools around the principles of asepsis.* FIG. 15: *In an emergency, surgeons could be great improvisers: this operating table was formed from two medicine panniers and their lids.* FIG. 16: *As operating theatres became restricted spaces, surgeons found new ways to demonstrate their techniques to students.*

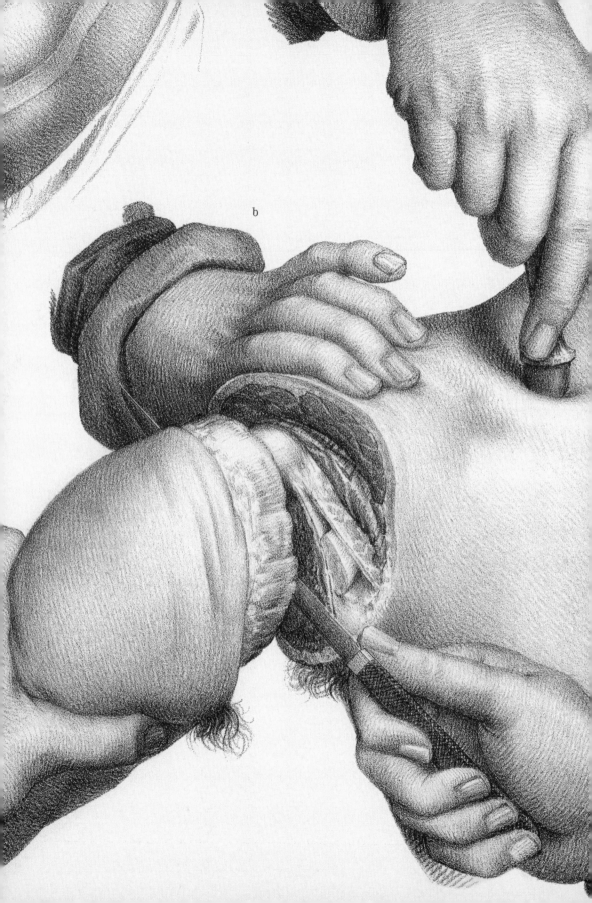

b

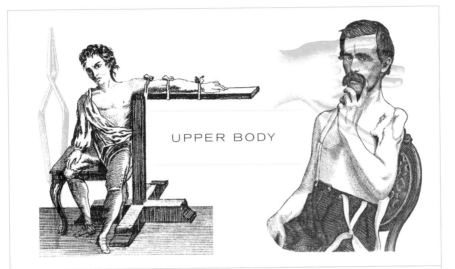

UPPER BODY

IV.

HANDS
& ARMS.

123

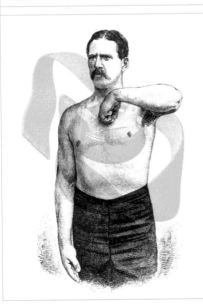

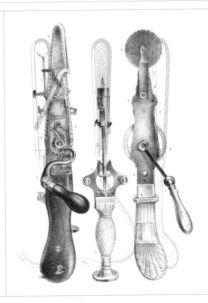

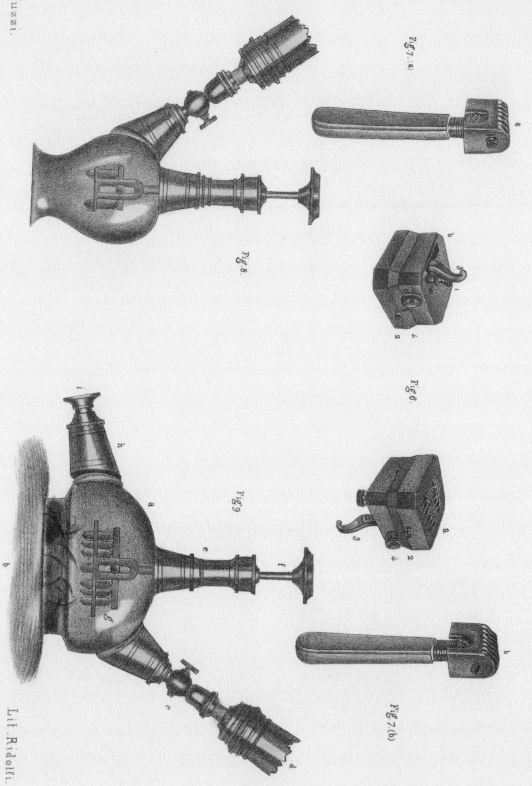

O.Muzzi.

Lit.Ridolfi.

Fig.7.(a)

Fig.8.

Fig.6.

Fig.5.

Fig.9.

Fig.7.(b)

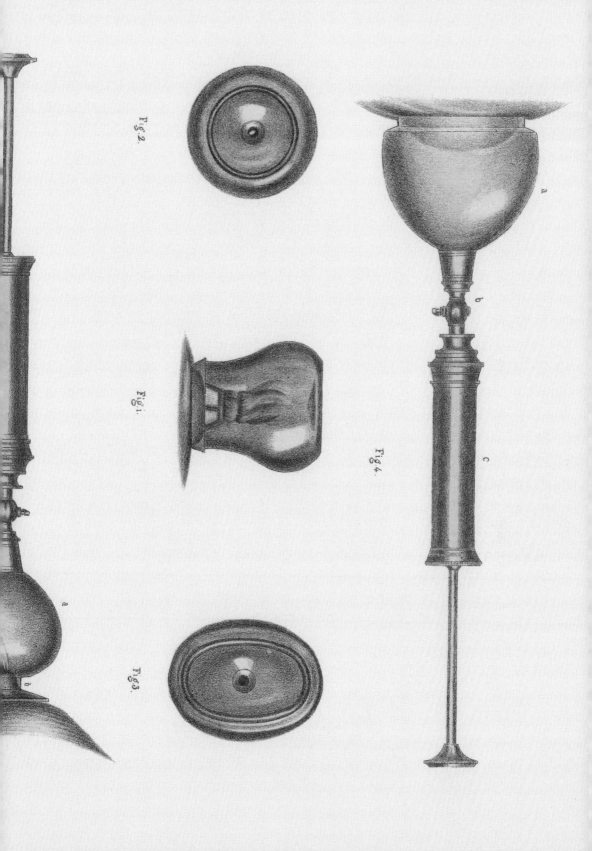

Fig. 2.

Fig. 1.

Fig. 4.

Fig. 3.

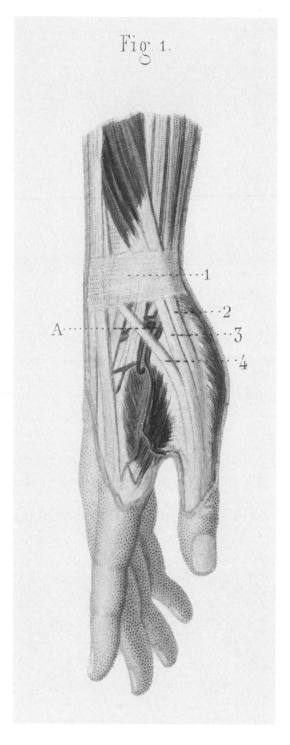

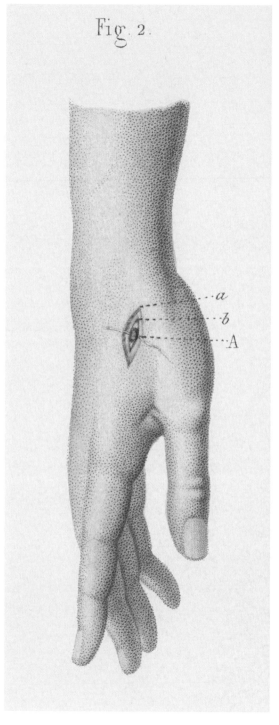

PREVIOUS: PAGE 122 | Circular amputation of the
arm at the shoulder. PAGES 124–125 | Instruments
for cupping and scarifying (and a breast pump).

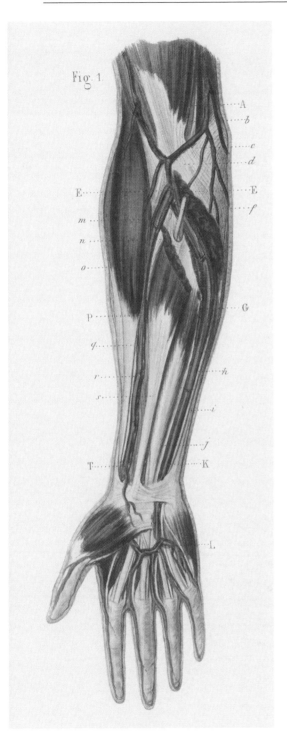

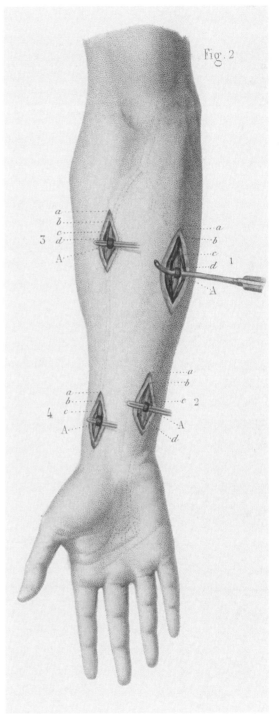

OPPOSITE: *(left)* Musculature and blood supply of the wrist and hand. *(right)* Sites for ligature of the radial artery.

ABOVE: *(left)* Musculature and blood supply of the lower arm, wrist and hand. *(right)* Sites for ligature of the ulnar and radial arteries.

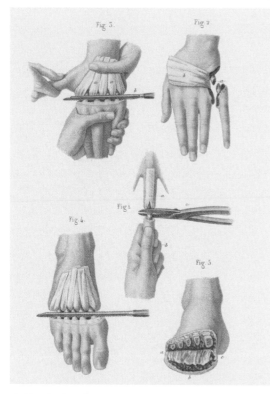

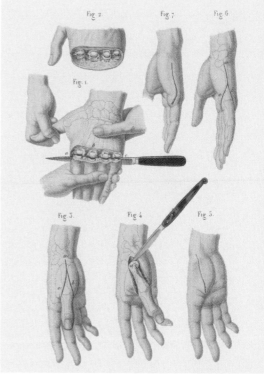

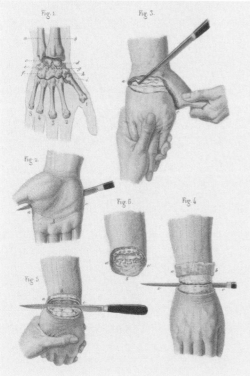

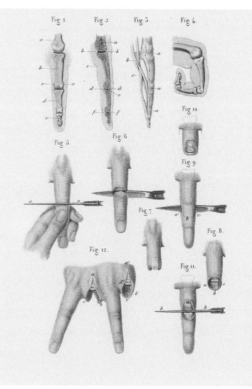

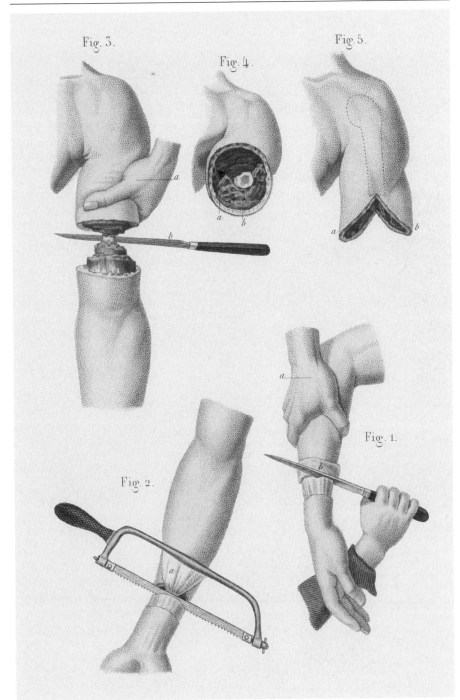

Fig. 3.

Fig. 4.

Fig. 5.

Fig. 1.

Fig. 2.

OPPOSITE: *(top left)* Amputation of the toes and fingers. *(top right)* Amputation of the fingers and thumb at the metacarpophalangeal joints. *(bottom left)* Amputation of the hand at the radiocarpal joint. *(bottom right)* Amputation of the fingers at the interphalangeal joints.

ABOVE: Amputation of the upper and lower arm.

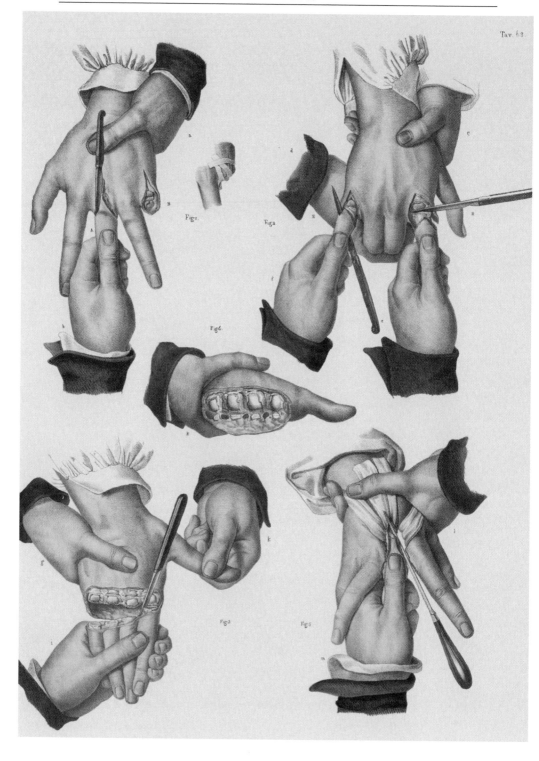

Tav. 68.

ABOVE: Techniques for amputation of the fingers.
OPPOSITE: Techniques for amputation of the fingers and thumb with the metacarpals.

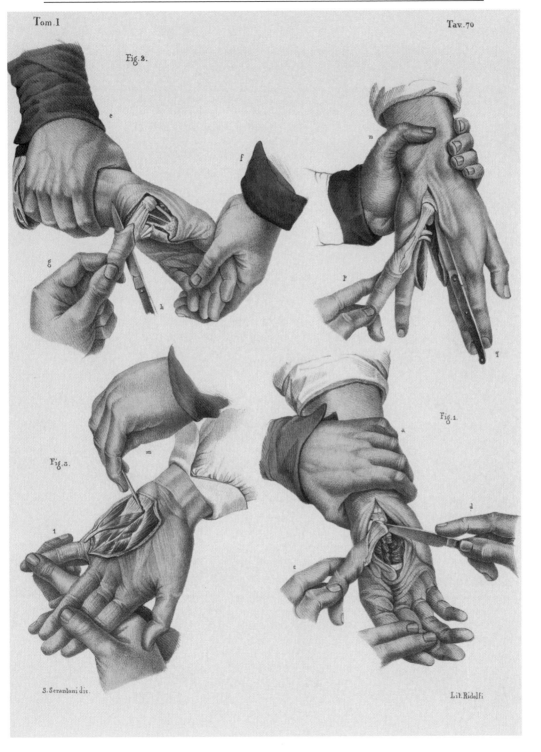

S. Serantoni dis.   Lit. Ridolfi

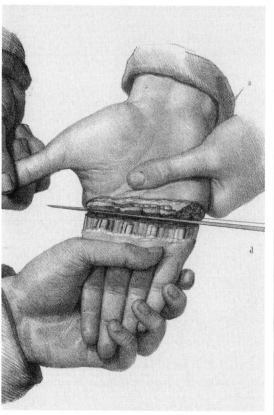

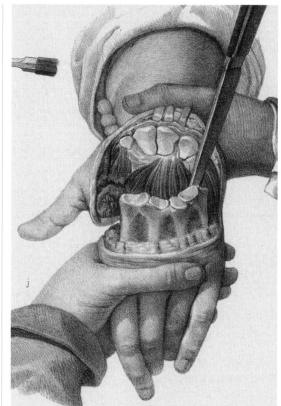

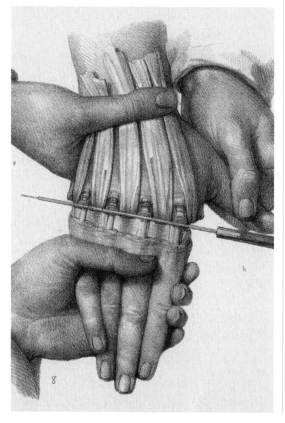

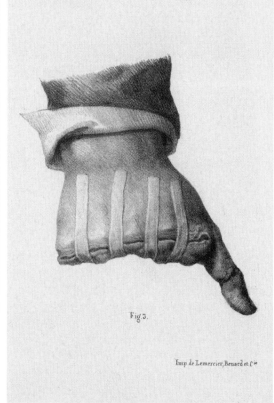

Fig 5.

Imp de Lemercier, Benard et Cie

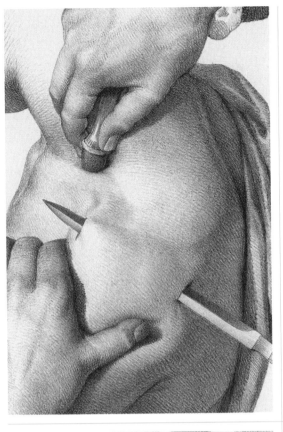

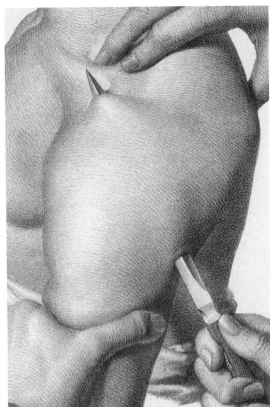

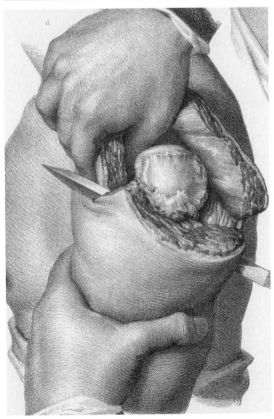

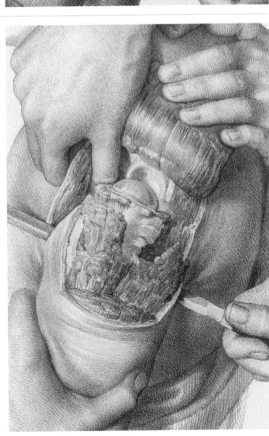

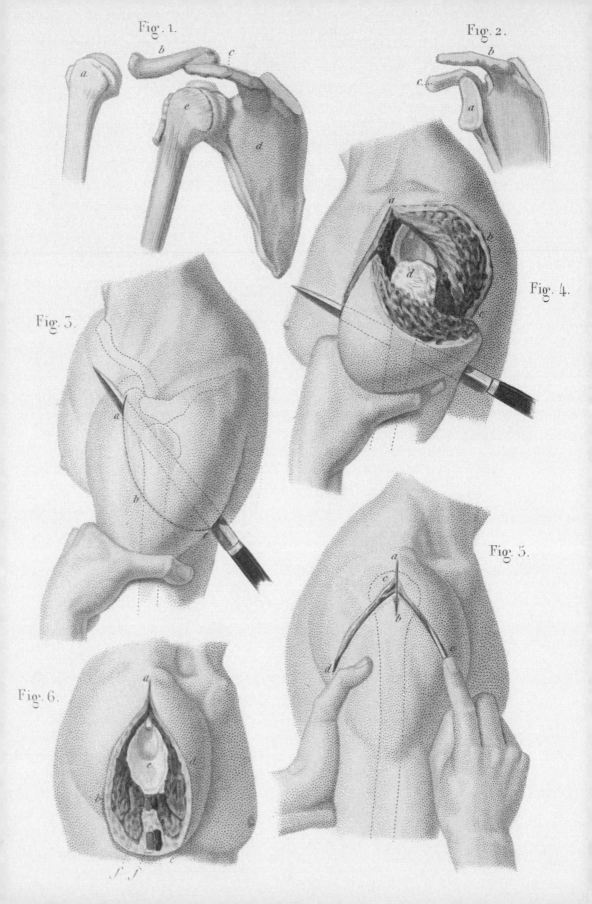

Fig. 1.

Fig. 2.

Fig. 3.

Fig. 4.

Fig. 5.

Fig. 6.

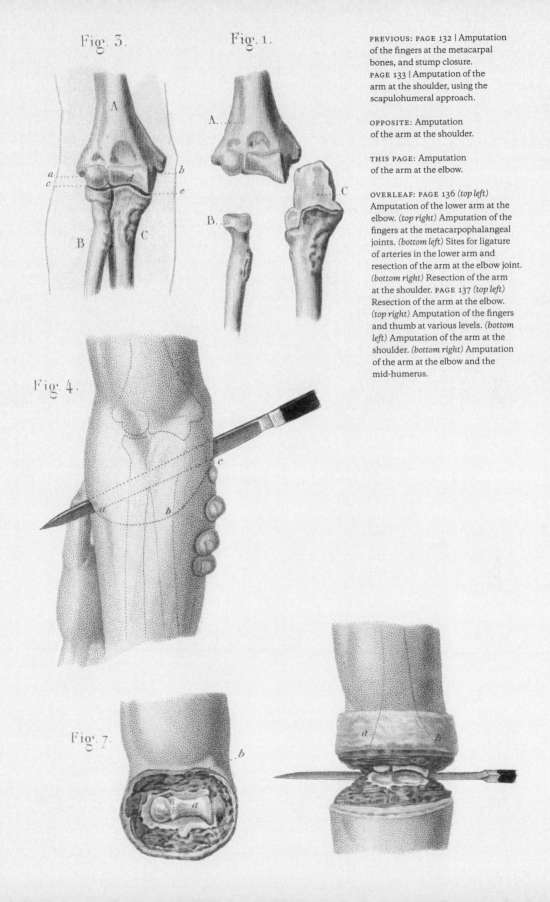

Fig. 3.　Fig. 1.

A

a
c
d
b
e

B　C

A

B

C

Fig. 4.

c
a
b

Fig. 7.

b

a

a

b

PREVIOUS: PAGE 132 | Amputation of the fingers at the metacarpal bones, and stump closure. PAGE 133 | Amputation of the arm at the shoulder, using the scapulohumeral approach.

OPPOSITE: Amputation of the arm at the shoulder.

THIS PAGE: Amputation of the arm at the elbow.

OVERLEAF: PAGE 136 (top left) Amputation of the lower arm at the elbow. (top right) Amputation of the fingers at the metacarpophalangeal joints. (bottom left) Sites for ligature of arteries in the lower arm and resection of the arm at the elbow joint. (bottom right) Resection of the arm at the shoulder. PAGE 137 (top left) Resection of the arm at the elbow. (top right) Amputation of the fingers and thumb at various levels. (bottom left) Amputation of the arm at the shoulder. (bottom right) Amputation of the arm at the elbow and the mid-humerus.

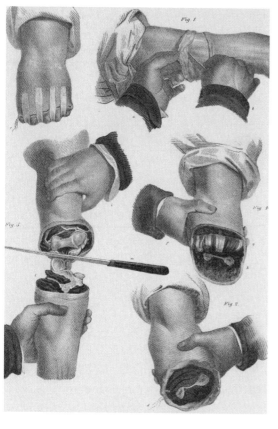

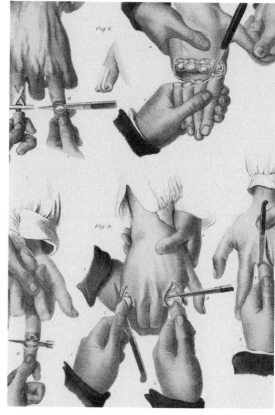

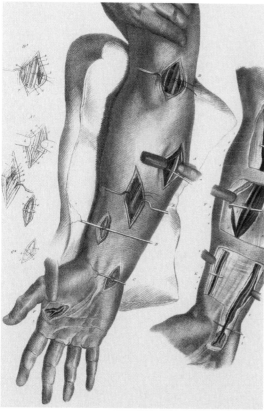

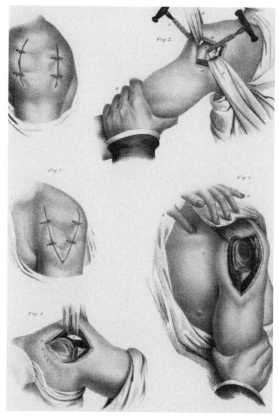

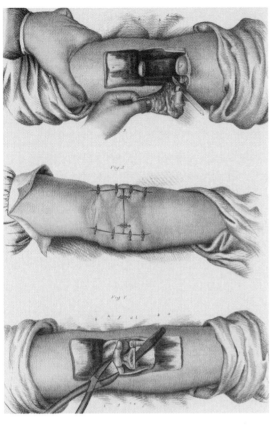

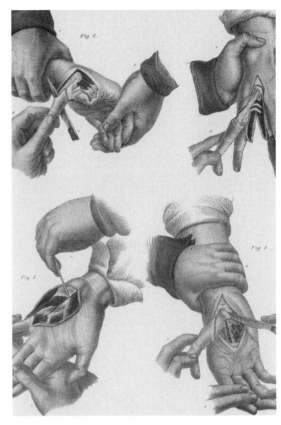

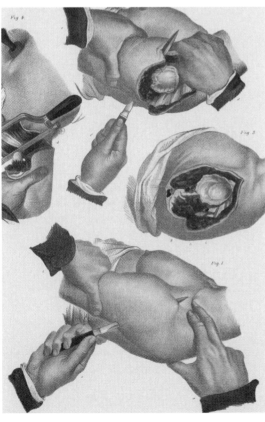

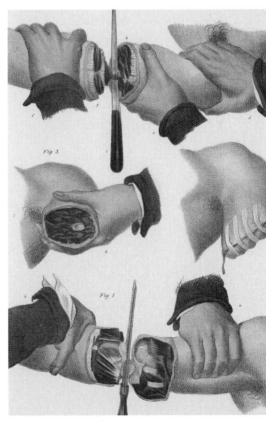

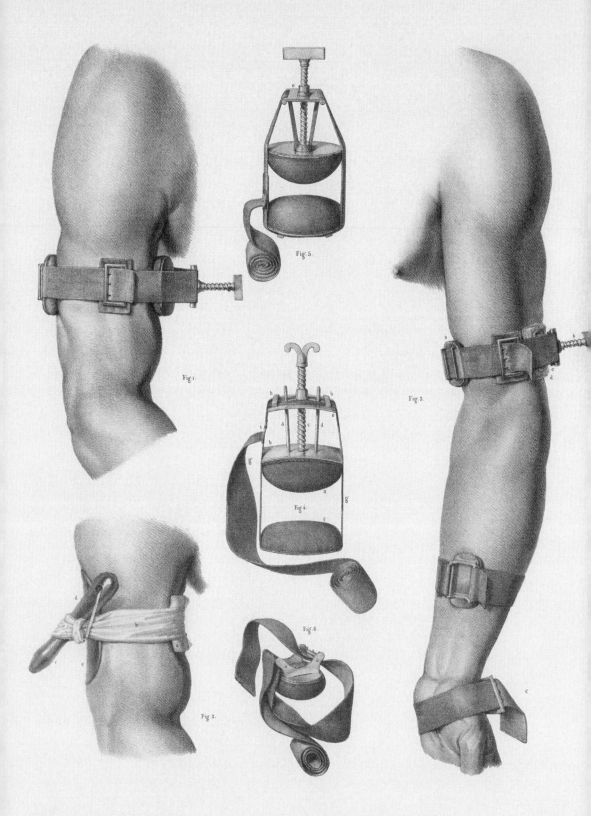

Fig 1.

Fig 2.

Fig. 3.

Fig. 4.

Fig. 5.

Fig. 6.

Dessiné par Léveillé
d'après nature par N.H. Jacob

Instruments de la Fabrique de M.r Charrière

Lith. de Lemercier, Benard et C.ie

Pl. 74.

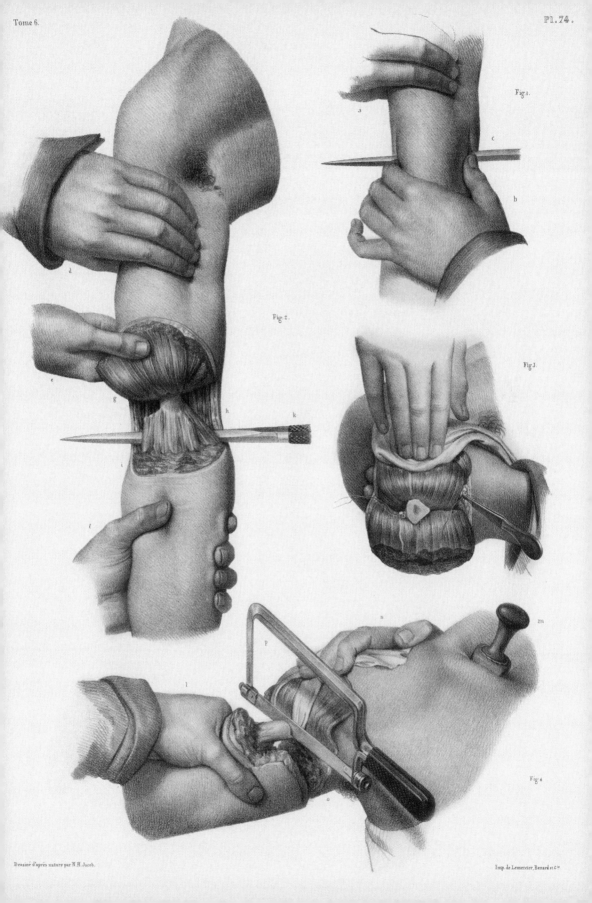

Fig. 1.

Fig. 2.

Fig. 3.

Fig. 4.

Dessiné d'après nature par N.H.Jacob.

Imp. de Lemercier, Benard et Cⁱᵉ.

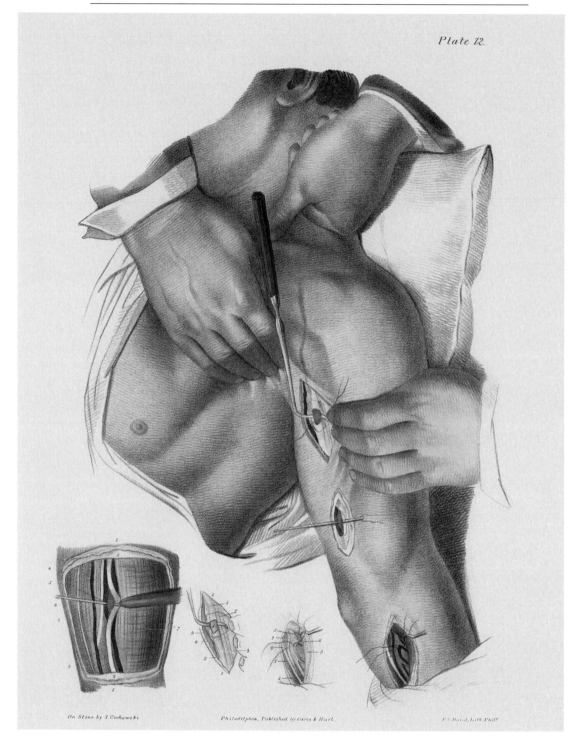

On Stone by S. Cichowski.   Philadelphia, Published by Carey & Hart.   P. S. Duval, lith. Phil?

PREVIOUS: PAGE 138 | Compression of the humeral, radial and ulnar arteries, to reduce blood loss during surgery. PAGE 139 | Amputation of the upper and lower arm.

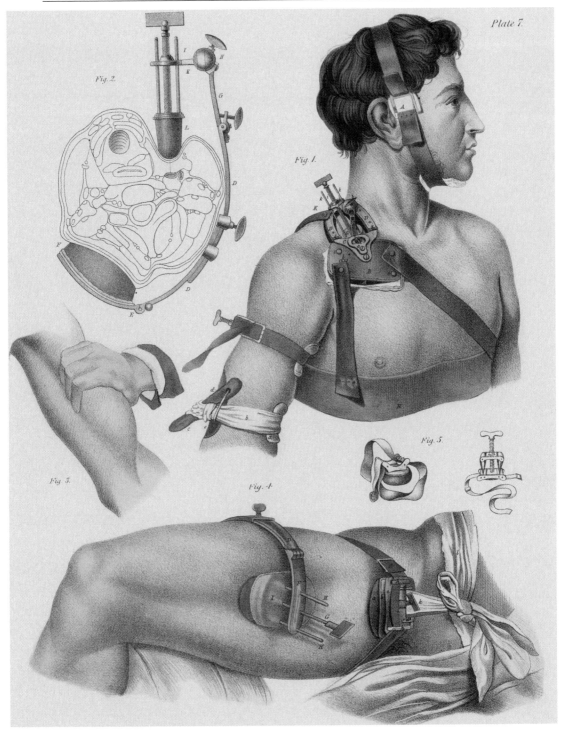

Fig. 2.

Fig. 1.

Plate 7.

Fig. 3.

Fig. 4.

Fig. 5.

OPPOSITE: Ligature of the humeral and ulnar arteries.
ABOVE: Compression of arteries in the arm and leg, to reduce blood loss during surgery.

MINISTERS OF HYGIENE: *Surgery & Nursing.*

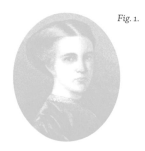

Fig. 1.

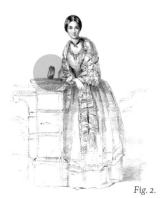

Fig. 2.

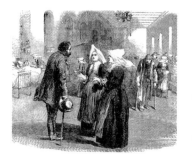

Fig. 3.

With only a handful of recorded exceptions in the southern European surgical tradition, the operating theatre was, historically, a male workspace. Surgeons, students and dressers were all men, and women might experience surgery only in the harrowing and subordinate role of patient. By 1900, women were working as theatre assistants, observing operations as students, and even—against the views of a majority of their male colleagues— beginning to operate independently as surgeons. The destruction of this male monopoly began with the mid nineteenth-century revolution in nursing.

Historians of nursing face the same difficulties as historians of surgery: we know something of nurses, what they wrote and what was written about them, but the daily practices of nurses and the outcomes of their work for patients are far harder to recover. What we can say, however, is that their work was not just a matter of practical care and cleanliness. Those trained in the style of nursing pioneered by Florence Nightingale also brought bourgeois codes of cleanliness and order into the often filthy and chaotic setting of large city hospitals. Along with anaesthesia and the discipline demanded by aseptic surgery, nursing reform turned hospitals into places where one might choose to undergo surgery, rather than be forced into it by poverty or accident.

Two cultural contexts underpinned nineteenth-century debates over nursing: the traditional role

of religious orders in hospital care, particularly in
Catholic countries, and the embedded presumption
that looking after the sick or vulnerable was
women's work, and lower-class women's work at
that. From 1836, a new institution brought these
two strands together with a fresh emphasis on
hygiene and the medical management of the sick.
At his Institute for Protestant Deaconesses at
Kaiserswerth in Germany, the Lutheran minister
Theodor Fliedner taught practical nursing,
wound dressing, ward management, childcare,
and the basics of pharmacy. His work gained a
reputation across Europe, and in 1840 the Quaker
prison reformer Elizabeth Fry established an
Institute of Nursing in London. As its name
suggests, Fliedner's school drew heavily on the
religious tradition of nursing, and though the
direct influence of Christianity declined during
the nineteenth century, such schools retained the
notion of nursing as a vocation, characterized by
obedience and service.

Histories of Victorian nursing tend to begin and
end with Florence Nightingale. With her wealthy,
well-connected and pious upbringing, her vision of
God at the age of seventeen, the protracted struggle
with her family over her wish to train under Fliedner
at Kaiserswerth, her brief but astonishingly intense
service reorganizing the Scutari hospital in the
Crimean War; and the second half of her long life as
the most tireless semi-invalid in history, establishing
British nursing as a respectable profession and
campaigning on a bewildering range of issues, her
story is well-told. In this sense it is misleading to
view Nightingale as merely a nursing reformer. Her
career as a ward nurse, such as it had been, ended
with Scutari, and the real key to her success was her
involvement in hospital logistics. She trained nurses,
certainly, and worked to improve the care of patients,
but she also took a close interest in the cleanliness
of the hospital, the supply of fresh linen, the quality
of food, and the collection of hard data on mortality
and efficiency.

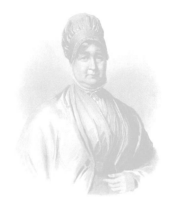

Fig. 4.

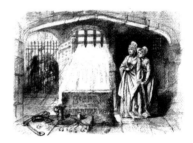

Fig. 5.

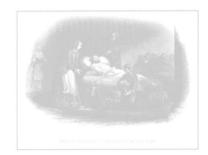

Fig. 6.

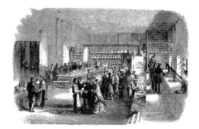

Fig. 7.

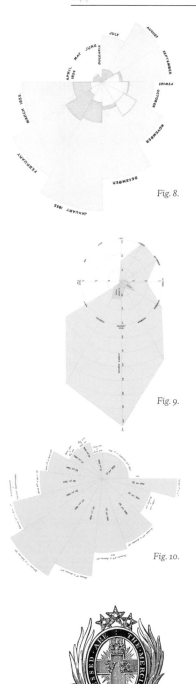

Fig. 8.

Fig. 9.

Fig. 10.

Fig. 11.

Returning to London in 1856, Nightingale found herself a national heroine, with her likeness printed everywhere on mass-market china and tea towels. She led a campaign to raise funds for a nursing school at the rebuilt St Thomas' Hospital; this opened in 1860 under her direction and with her *Notes on Nursing*, published the previous year, as its textbook. For Nightingale, nursing was no longer a talent that came naturally to women as a consequence of their gender.

Modern hospitals required nurses with up-to-date knowledge, practical experience and a professional attitude. Nightingale set out to create a generation of 'training matrons' who would take her model to every corner of the British Empire. Her ideas also gained influence during the American Civil War, through the work of Dorothea Dix, superintendent of the United States Army Nurses, and Clara Barton, founder of the American Red Cross.

Through the second half of the nineteenth century the number of nurses working in Britain rose dramatically: fewer than 1,000 in 1861 became around 70,000 by 1901. Though a majority of these new nurses never held a hospital post, almost all would have spent time as students on hospital wards, and Nightingale-style hospital nursing became the gold standard of practice. We can see this in 'The Florence Nightingale Pledge', a version of the Hippocratic Oath written by the American nursing reformer Lystra E. Gretter in 1893:

> *I solemnly pledge myself before God and in the presence of this assembly, to pass my life in purity and to practice my profession faithfully. I will abstain from whatever is deleterious and mischievous, and will not take or knowingly administer any harmful drug. I will do all in my power to maintain and elevate the standard of my profession, and will hold in confidence all personal matters committed to my keeping and all family affairs coming to my knowledge in the practice*

*of my calling. With loyalty will I endeavor to
aid the physician in his work, and devote myself
to the welfare of those committed to my care.*

Over a couple of generations, nursing acquired
a framework of professional and regulatory bodies:
the British (later Royal) Nursing Association
in 1887, and the Nursing Register and General
Nursing Council, created on the lines of the
Medical Register and the General Medical Council,
in 1919. One way to track the rising status of nurses
is through the ways in which they were paid. Before
Nightingale's reforms, nursing was generally treated
as a form of casual labour, with nurses paid by the
case or by the week. By the end of the nineteenth
century hospital nurses worked within a structured
system of employment, with regular (if modest)
wages, and the appearance of nursing agencies (like
those for secretaries or governesses) showed that
nursing was becoming a respectable occupation
for the daughters of the middle classes.

For young women raised in the restricted sphere
of the late Victorian bourgeois household, nursing
offered a chance to apply their skills in household
management and an outlet for their ingrained
sense of charitable Christian duty. Emotional and
sexual duties aside, the tasks allotted to a middle-
class housewife were not far from that which a
hospital matron would be expected to undertake
for a consultant surgeon. Both would supervise
the work of servants, ensure a reliable supply of
food and clean linen, and provide an efficient and
supportive backdrop for the work of professional
men. Nightingale nurses were taught anatomy
and physiology not in order to give them an
independent clinical perspective, but to make them
more efficient and reliable carers—a role enforced
by matrons, who exercised as much control over
nurses on their wards as consultants did over
their students.

The changing of antiseptic dressings gave nurses
their first role in the management of surgical cases

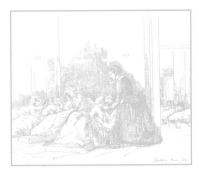

Fig. 12.

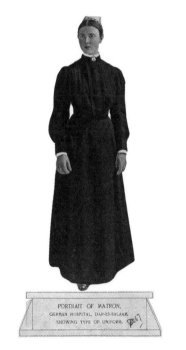

PORTRAIT OF MATRON,
GERMAN HOSPITAL, DAR-ES-SALAAM,
SHOWING TYPE OF UNIFORM.

Fig. 13.

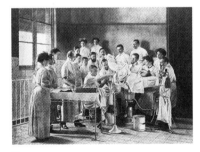

Fig. 14.

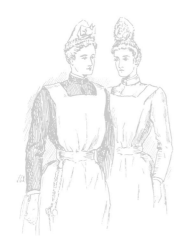

Fig. 15.

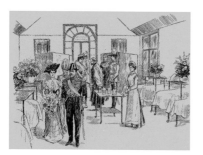

Fig. 16.

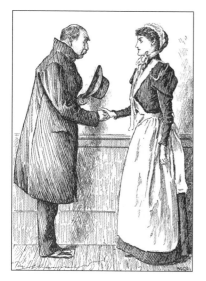

Fig. 17.

and an entrée to the operating theatre. Anaesthesia had made the operating theatre a place of quiet science rather than violent physical assault on a conscious patient, and hence a setting in which the Victorian concept of feminine sensibility would be less vulnerable to offence. The first theatre nurses were assistants in the rituals of surgical antisepsis, turning the traditionally female tasks of cleaning, swabbing and stitching into clinical necessities. Nightingale herself appears never to have entered an operating theatre, and her nurses received no detailed education in theatre practice, but surgeons began to train their own nurses on the job, in the process building deep professional—and sometimes emotional—bonds.

As the relationship between surgery, science and the hospital was remade over the late nineteenth century, so new forms of nursing altered patients' experiences of hospital care. This might be practical—a new emphasis, for example, on 'nursing sightlines', so that a matron at her desk could see every patient on her ward. But patients, surgeons and nurses also found themselves enrolled in a new hierarchy, overseen by bureaucrats and founded on new ideas of scientific management and efficiency. Nurses were taken up as symbols of what hospitals were becoming—clean, progressive, respectable—and the image of a beautiful young woman in a starched uniform, watching at the bedside of a patient, became a staple of fundraising campaigns for new wards or equipment. These avatars of modernity occupied a curiously equivocal position: as members of a profession, but possessors of a vocation, they were the heirs to a long Christian tradition, and the handmaidens of the new era of scientific surgery.

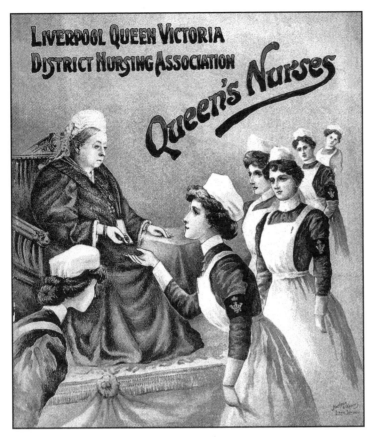

Fig. 18.

FIG. 1: *Elizabeth Garrett Anderson (1836-1917), the first woman in Britain to qualify as a physician and surgeon.*
FIG. 2: *The young Florence Nightingale and her pet owl, Athena.* FIG. 3: *Religious orders took traditional responsibility for providing nurses, such as these Sisters of Charity at a Turkish hospital during the Crimean War.*
FIG. 4: *Elizabeth Fry (1780-1845), prison reformer and founder of London's Institute of Nursing.* FIG. 5: *Fry visiting Newgate Prison as part of her campaign to reform British prisons.* FIG. 6: *A romantically idealized vision of Nightingale's work at the Scutari Hospital during the Crimean War.* FIG. 7: *Nightingale worked with the French chef Alexis Soyer at Scutari, and his hospital kitchen (shown here) proved popular with patients.* FIG. 8: *Nightingale used these 'coxcomb diagrams'—pie charts—as a vivid demonstration of British mortality rates in the Crimea.*
FIG. 9: *This 'coxcomb diagram' compares mortality rates from wounds, infectious diseases, and other causes among British troops in the Crimea in 1854-56.* FIG. 10: *This 'coxcomb diagram' compares mortality rates at the Scutari and Kulali hospitals in 1854-55.* FIG. 11: *This brooch—the 'Nightingale Jewel'—was designed by Prince Albert and presented by Queen Victoria to Florence Nightingale, in lieu of an official medal or decoration, on her return from the Crimea in 1856.* FIG. 12: *During the Crimean War, British newspapers made much of Nightingale's exploits as 'the Lady with the Lamp'—an image captured in this 1854 lithograph.* FIG. 13: *By the late nineteenth century, Nightingale matrons—capable, austere, no-nonsense—were working in hospitals around the world, in this case the General Hospital in Dar-es-Salaam.* FIG. 14: *In the second half of the nineteenth century, female nurses began to replace male assistants in European operating theatres, such as this one in Paris.* FIG. 15: *Nursing uniforms such as these, for St George's Hospital in London, were designed to convey an impression of cleanliness, order and efficiency.*
FIG. 16: *King Edward VII and Queen Alexandra visiting the Royal Victoria Hospital in Belfast in 1903, attended by uniformed nurses.* FIG. 17: *'If ever there was a fallen hangel, you're one!' A cured patient pays an ambivalent compliment to his nurse in this cartoon by George du Maurier (1834-1896).* FIG. 18: *By the end of the nineteenth century nursing had gained respectability and—as this booklet from the Liverpool Queen Victoria District Nursing Association shows—royal patronage.*

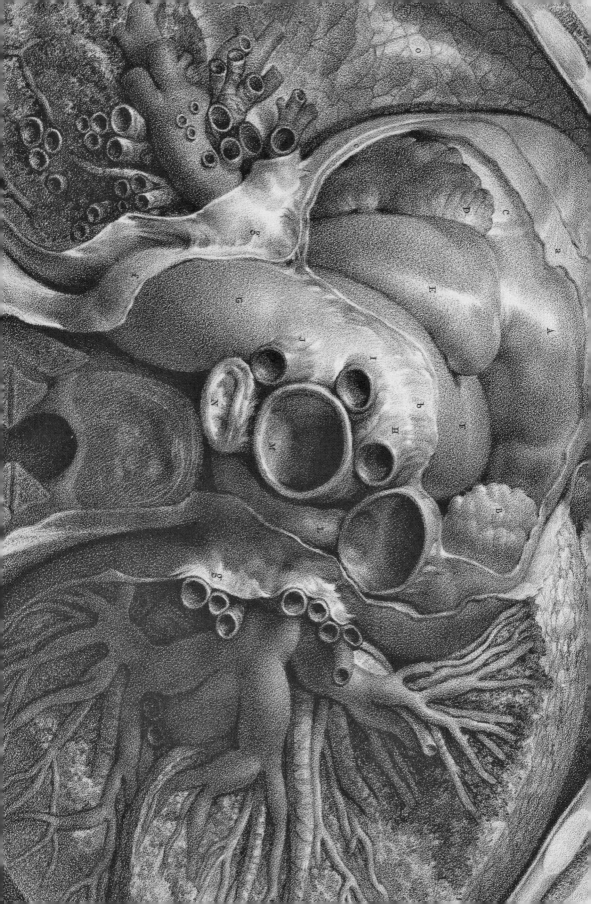

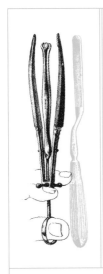
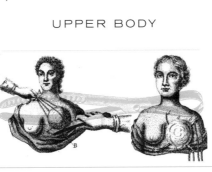

UPPER BODY

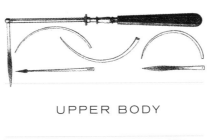

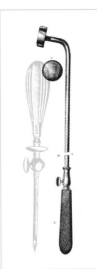

V. ## *CHEST.* 149

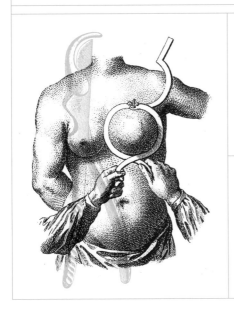

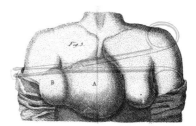

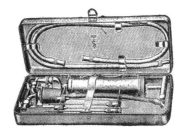

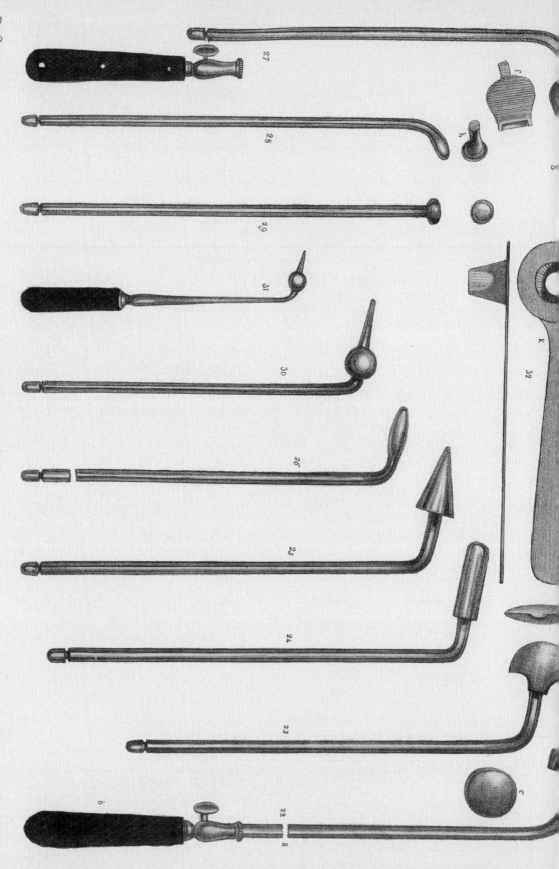

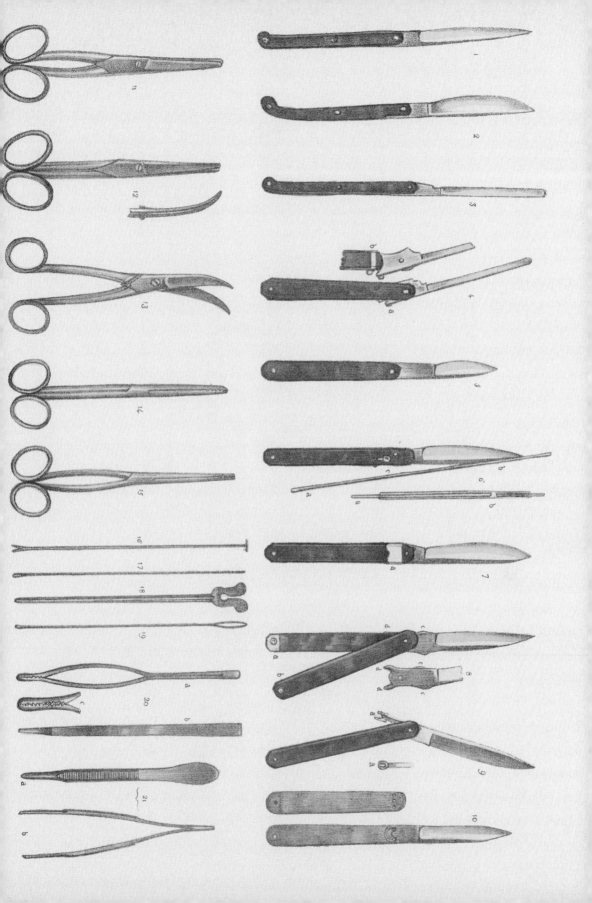

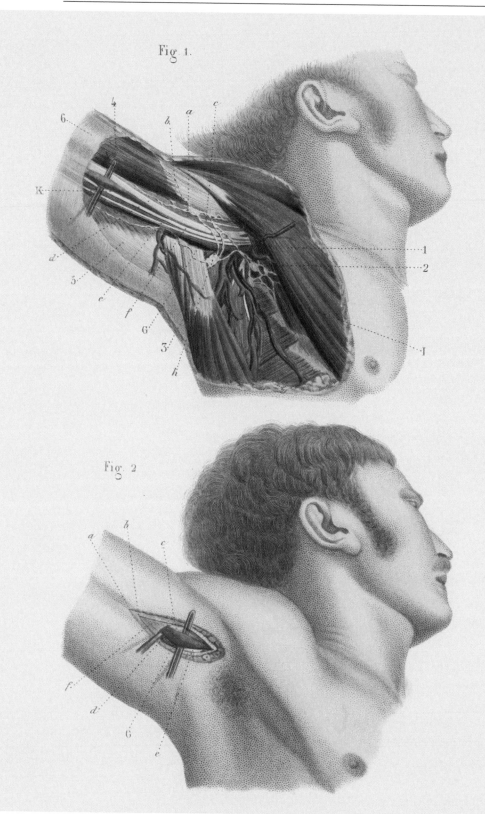

Fig. 1.

Fig. 2

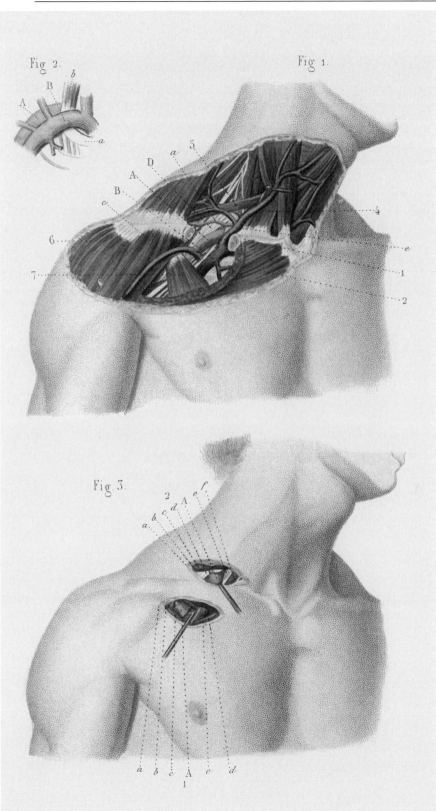

Fig 2.

Fig 1.

Fig 3.

PREVIOUS:
PAGE 148 | Dissection
of the chest, showing
the great vessels of the
heart and the vessels
of the lungs. PAGES
150-151 | A selection
of instruments used
for cauterization,
incision and wound
dressing.

OPPOSITE: Anatomy
of the armpit, and
ligature of the axillary
armpit.

THIS PAGE: Anatomy
of the neck and
shoulder, and ligature
of the axillary and
subclavian arteries.

OVERLEAF: *(left)*
Dissection of a seated
man, showing the
aorta and the major
arteries of the thorax
and abdomen. *(right)*
Dissection of the
thorax, showing the
relative position of
the lungs, heart, and
primary blood vessels.

Pl. 25.

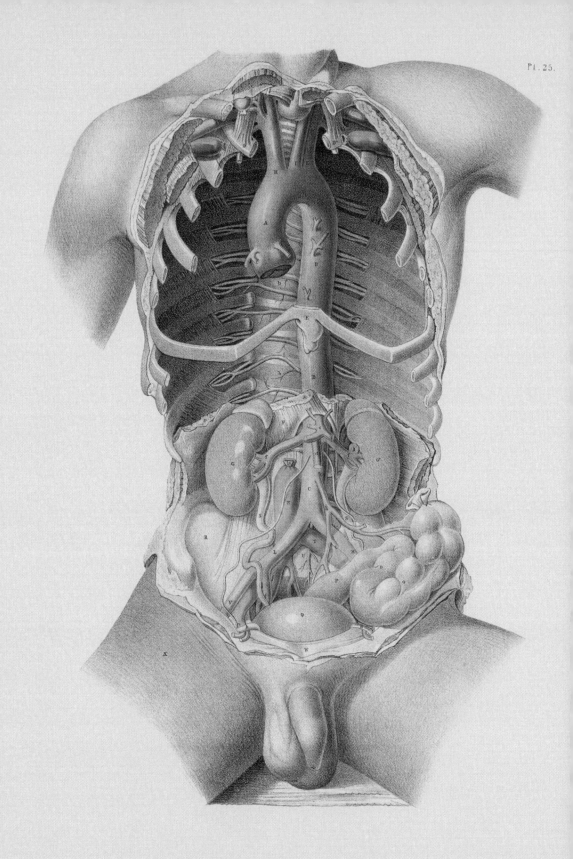

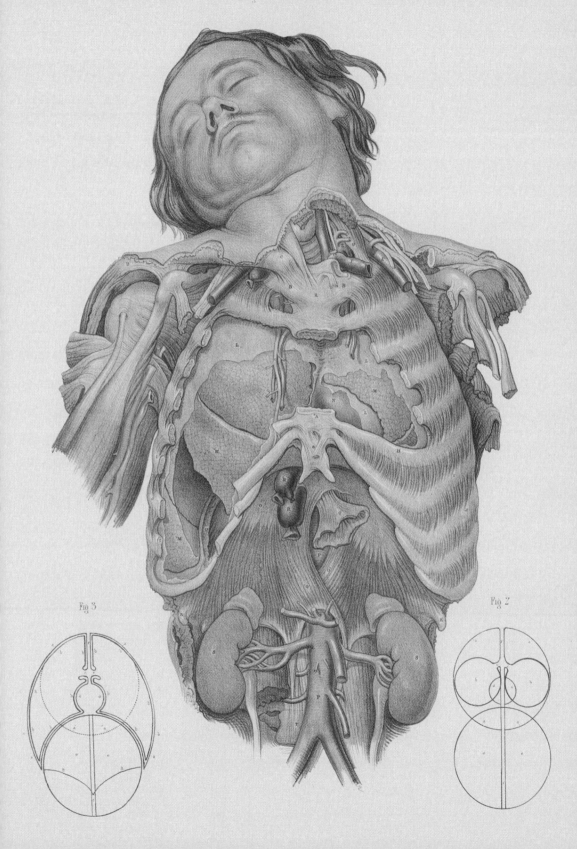

Fig 1

Fig 3

Fig 2

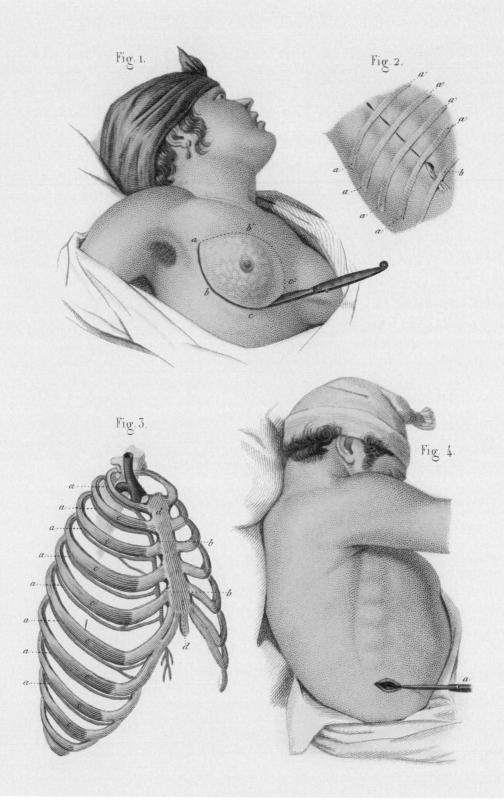

Fig. 1.

Fig. 2.

Fig. 3.

Fig. 4.

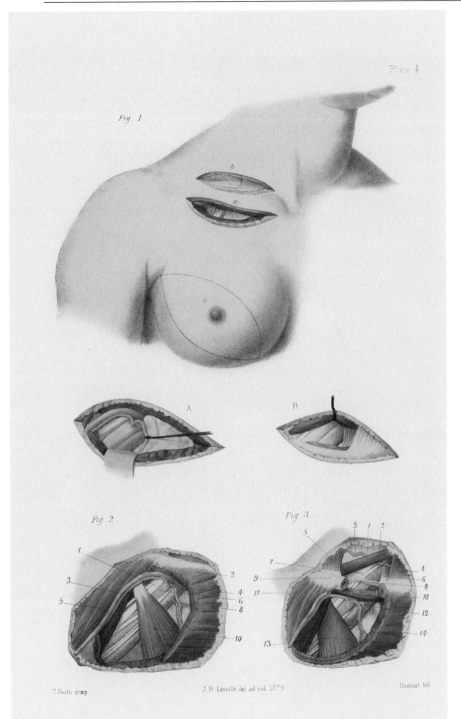

Plate 4

fig. 1.

b

a

c

A

B

Fig. 2.

1
3
5

2
4
6
8

10

Fig. 3.

5

3 1 2

7

9

11

4
6
8
10

12

14

13

C. Heath prasp   J. B. Léveillé del ad nat 1875   Hanhart lith.

OPPOSITE: Technique for mastectomy, wound closure, anatomy of intercostal muscles, and drainage of empyema.

THIS PAGE: Ligature of the axillary and subclavian arteries, excision of the breast, and anatomy of axilla and shoulder.

OVERLEAF: *(left)* Excision of breast and wound dressing. *(right)* Surgical drainage of empyema.

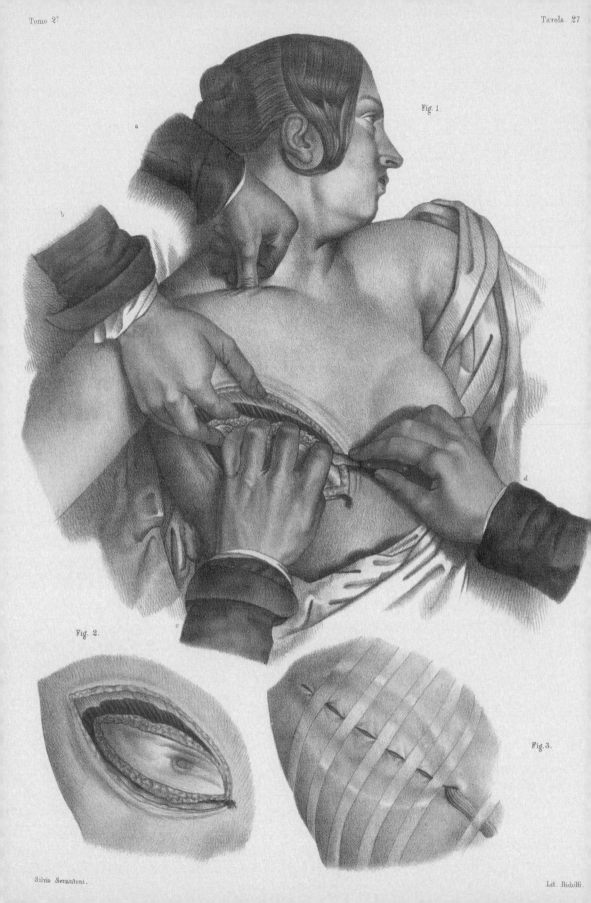

Fig. 1.

Fig. 2.

Fig. 3.

Silvio Serantoni.   Lit. Ridolfi.

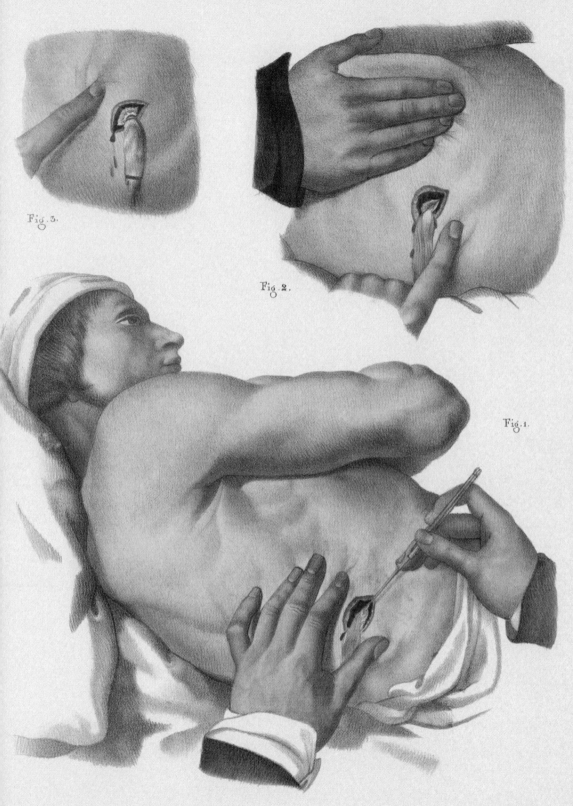

THE SMART OF THE KNIFE: *Surgery & War.*

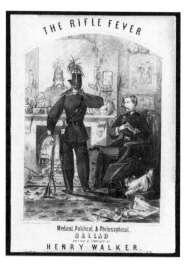

Fig. 1.

[1] Roger Cooter, 'War and modern medicine', in William Bynum and Roy Porter (eds), *Companion Encyclopaedia of the History of Medicine*, (London, England: Routledge, 1993), 1536–63.

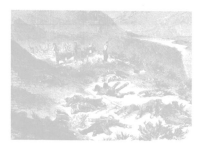

Fig. 2.

Reflecting in 1858 on his Crimean War service, the Scottish army surgeon George Macleod struck a note of optimism:

> *A great war, in short, is a great epoch in the onward march of surgical science, when the slowly elaborated teachings of civil life are tested on a grand scale in the presence of representatives from every school.*

Underlying Macleod's stirring Victorian rhetoric is the proposal that war has been an unfortunate but effective stimulus of medical and surgical progress—an argument expressed repeatedly in the writings of nineteenth-century military surgeons. Roger Cooter has observed that histories of medicine and war tend to be preoccupied with 'great men, great battles and great technical achievements'.[1] Looking beyond these concerns, we get a very different impression of the meaning of war for surgeons like Macleod. In the eighteenth and early nineteenth centuries war was, for most European nations and in most cases, something that a fairly small army of private soldiers went abroad to do. Civilians back home might hear of great victories in news-sheets or ballads, and see limbless ex-servicemen begging at street corners, but the business of fighting, and of dealing with its immediate aftermath, took place in a different sphere. The American Civil War and the Franco-Prussian War heralded a new

kind of conflict, one in which entire populations
contributed to the war effort and, all too often,
suffered and died like soldiers. In their encounters
with this new and terrible 'total war', both surgery
and society were transformed.

As we saw in the introduction, many eighteenth-
century surgeons served with armies or navies, and
in this role they also took general responsibility
for the health of soldiers or—especially—sailors.
In 1805, at the time of the Battle of Trafalgar, the
Royal College of Surgeons recommended that
a naval surgeon's supply chest should contain
saws, screw tourniquets and bone nippers, but
also camphor, ipecac, opium, and senna. Stormy
weather could mean that a ship's hatches were
battened down for weeks on end, with supplies
rotting as seawater trickled into the hold, and
outbreaks of fever might well be blamed on the
stagnant shipboard atmosphere. With no specific
treatments, captains and surgeons fumigated ships
with brimstone or gunpowder, and kept crews
occupied with swabbing the decks.

Back on land, early modern states were taking
an interest in providing care for sick or wounded
servicemen. London's Royal Chelsea Hospital
and Royal Hospital for Seamen, and the Hôtel
des Invalides in Paris, were founded in the late
seventeenth century to care for aged or permanently
disabled veterans. The Edinburgh Royal Infirmary,
opened in 1752, had separate military wards for
soldiers and seamen, and Hampshire's Royal
Hospital Haslar, Britain's first dedicated naval
hospital and at the time the largest brick structure in
the country, received a charter from George I in 1753.
Half a century later, as Napoleon threatened Britain's
naval defences, the government funded a regius
professorship of military surgery at Edinburgh. Its
first occupant, the surgeon John Thompson, offered
six-month courses to surgeons working in the army,
the navy, or—a mark of British colonial reach—the
Indian Health Service. Notes taken by one of his
students give us a flavour of Thompson's syllabus:

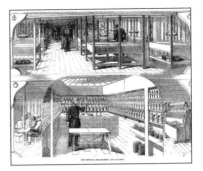

Fig. 3.

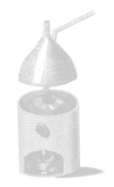

Fig. 4.

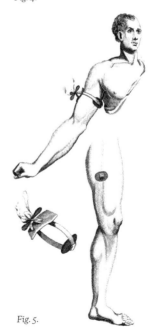

Fig. 5.

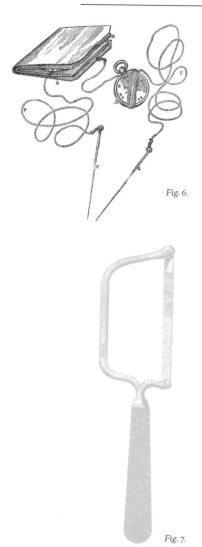

Fig. 6.

Fig. 7.

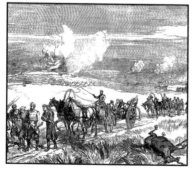

Fig. 8.

Gunshot wounds—consideration of various kinds of missiles; initial management; extraction of foreign bodies… Dressing of wounds, Contused wounds, Penetration wounds, Tetanus, Injuries of the head—scalp, cranium, depressed fractures, Wounds of the brain, Concussion, Wounds of the eyes, cheeks, chest, thorax, intestines, extremities.

Battlefield surgery such as this was, ironically, a process of rendering injured men unfit to fight— either in the short term, while wounds healed, or in the long term, with the loss of a limb. And the martial ideal of heroic bravado was more fragile than soldiers might care to admit. Facing the amputation of his foot after a battle in 1814, Sergeant Thomas Jackson of the Coldstream Guards downed a pint of wine and greeted his surgeon with a joke. But the saw was blunt, and stuck in his tibia 'as a bad saw would when sawing a green stick'. Tying off severed blood vessels and dressing the wound proved even more painful, and this battle-hardened and courageous soldier later wrote that his attendants had been 'not very nice about hurting one'.

By the mid nineteenth century, military surgeons were facing problems that went far beyond the individual suffering of men such as Jackson. Industrialization, imperialism, mass transport and mass communication were changing the nature of warfare. High-velocity bullets caused devastating wounds, and fragments from high-explosive shells drove shrapnel and earth deep into soldiers' bodies, making debridement and infection control near-impossible. Trench warfare—an established tactic by the time of the American Civil War—could cause intractable problems such as trench foot, and also altered the psychology of combat. Troops served long watches in dugouts, all the while knowing they could meet a sudden, violent and impersonal death from shellfire or a sniper. It seems hardly surprising that these conflicts produced the first large-scale reports of what would come to be called shell shock.

Behind the lines, the sheer scale of total war proved the greatest challenge. Large, fast-moving armies required mobile, flexible supply lines for food, ammunition and kit. On top of that, the numbers of men killed in battles—a grim parody of industrial mass production—called for resilient systems of evacuation, triage, treatment and repatriation. Early debates over the place of surgery in mechanized warfare revolved around the provision of anaesthetics. At the outbreak of the Crimean War, the British army's chief medical officer, Sir John Hall, told his officers that 'the smart of the knife is a powerful stimulant and it is better to hear a man bawl lustily than to see him sink silently into the grave'. Two themes are at work in this much-derided remark: first, the question of whether anaesthetics would make soldiers less tolerant of pain and therefore more cowardly; and second, whether shocked or severely wounded soldiers were more vulnerable to the acknowledged risks of chloroform.

Despite Hall's opposition, chloroform was issued to British surgeons and used for surgery at large hospitals such as Scutari, though its use in the field tended to reflect the attitudes of individual surgeons and the simple fact of its availability. By the end of the war, French surgeons were reporting more than 25,000 anaesthetics given to wounded soldiers, apparently without a single fatality, and Hall reversed his view, recommending it for all battlefield surgery. During the American Civil War, surgeons on both sides used chloroform (a highly sought-after item of war booty), and when General Thomas 'Stonewall' Jackson had his arm amputated after being shot by his own troops at the Battle of Chancellorsville, he described chloroform as 'the most delightful physical sensation I ever experienced'.

Arguments over battlefield anaesthesia were a microcosm of larger questions about the shifting nature of surgery. For centuries, the standard response to limb trauma had been quick amputation,

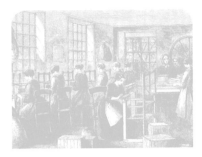

Fig. 9.

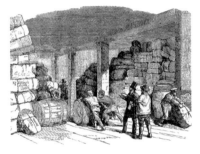

Fig. 10.

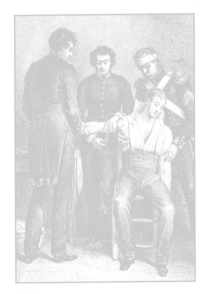

Fig. 11.

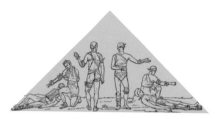

Fig. 12.

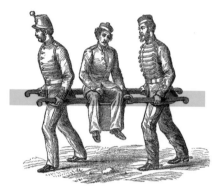

Fig. 13.

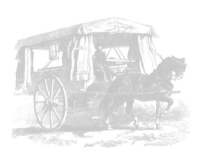

Fig. 14.

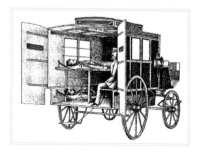

Fig. 15.

as attested by accounts of severed limbs heaped up outside field hospitals. Military surgeons had gained great skill at cutting off legs and arms, but were they too keen? Would it be better to excise and conserve, or would the extra time taken result in more fatalities? And did conservative surgery actually preserve any real function? The English surgeon Edward Wrench put it bluntly:

> *No arm is much better for a soldier than an arm of little use, for the first he gets a shilling a day pension whereas for the latter he gets nothing, but is just turned out as unfit for service.*

Military innovations such as ambulances began to appear in civilian life, while paramedical organizations such as the Red Cross and the St John Ambulance Brigade (along with the Salvation Army and Baden-Powell's Boy Scouts) adopted military uniforms, ranks and parades, and surgeons and physicians began to use battlefield metaphors in talking about their work. In part this reflected the rise of bacteriology, which took disease as an enemy to be defeated rather than an imbalance to be corrected.

'Painkiller' first appeared in English in 1845, and around the same time case notes begin to include descriptions of pain as 'shooting', or comparisons with the bursting of shells. Surgeons became 'soldiers for humanity'; new drugs were 'magic bullets'; and these comparisons were hard to resist. Writing at the end of the First World War, the Scottish military surgeon H. M. W. Gray warned his readers that:

> *Antiseptics affect bacteria embedded in [wounds] no more than shrapnel or rifle fire dislodges the Hun lurking in fortified dugouts.*

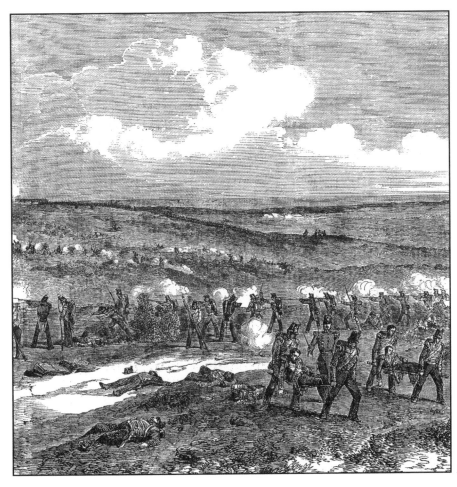

Fig. 16.

FIG. 1: *Battlefield injuries could be horrific, but many more British troops died in the Crimea from infections and diseases than from wounds.* FIG. 2: *'The Rifle Fever': patriotic songs and journalism presented a deeply romanticized and heroic vision of modern warfare.* FIG. 3: *During the Crimean War (1853-1856), HMS Melbourne served as a floating hospital and operating theatre.* FIG. 4: *Naval surgeons traditionally held responsibility for the general health of their crews, and fumigators such as this one were a common way of cleansing the air below deck.* FIG. 5: *In the aftermath of a battle, naval or military surgery was usually a matter of rapid amputation on a terrible scale.* FIG. 6: *This simple electric battery and circuit, designed in 1875, was one solution to the problem of locating deeply embedded lead bullets.* FIG. 7: *With saws such as this and long, sharp knives, battlefield surgeons could amputate limbs within minutes.* FIG. 8: *The American Civil War (1861-1865) highlighted the problems of modern mass warfare—not least, the matter of moving the wounded safely away from the battlefield.* FIG. 9: *Women in an English factory made large quantities of lint dressings for the British Army in the Crimea.* FIG. 10: *Efforts to improve conditions for those wounded in the Crimea were hampered by the long chain of logistical support stretching back to Britain, more than a thousand miles away.* FIG. 11: *Even battle-hardened soldiers could be taken aback by the pain of amputation.* FIG. 12: *From the late nineteenth century, field dressings such as these became part of soldiers' basic kit.* FIG. 13: *Soldiers wounded on a battlefield might receive immediate first-aid and evacuation from their comrades.* FIG. 14: *Horse-drawn ambulances such as these were an improvised response to the high rates of British battlefield casualties in the Crimea.* FIG. 15: *Back in civilian life, hospitals were fairly quick to adopt military innovations such as this ambulance, designed for the Metropolitan Asylums Board.* FIG. 16: *No medical or surgical innovations could disguise the fact that nineteenth-century battlefields—Sevastopol, during the Crimean War, is shown here—could be confusing, brutal and painful places.*

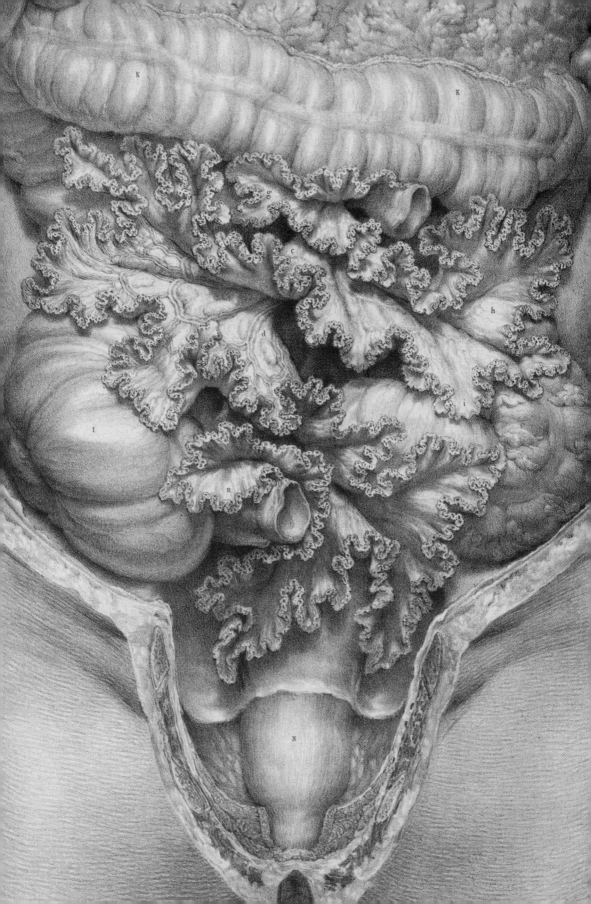

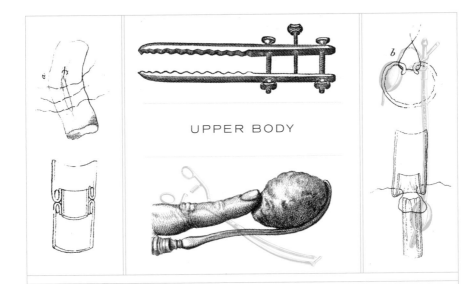

UPPER BODY

VI

ABDOMEN.

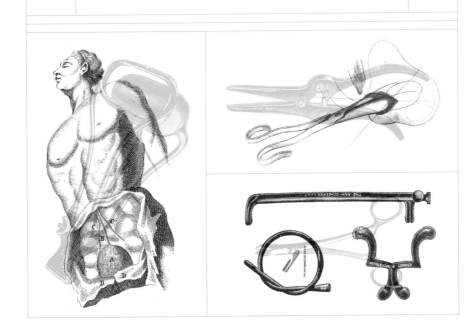

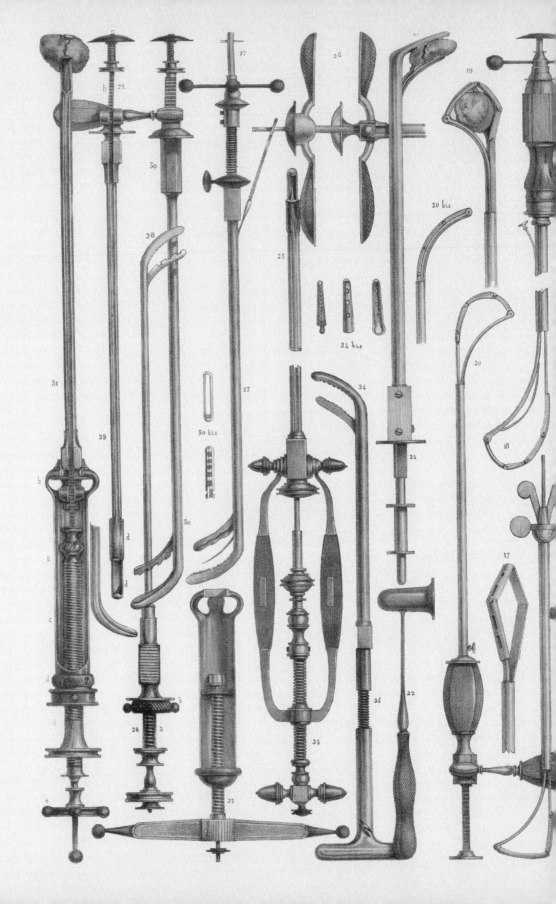

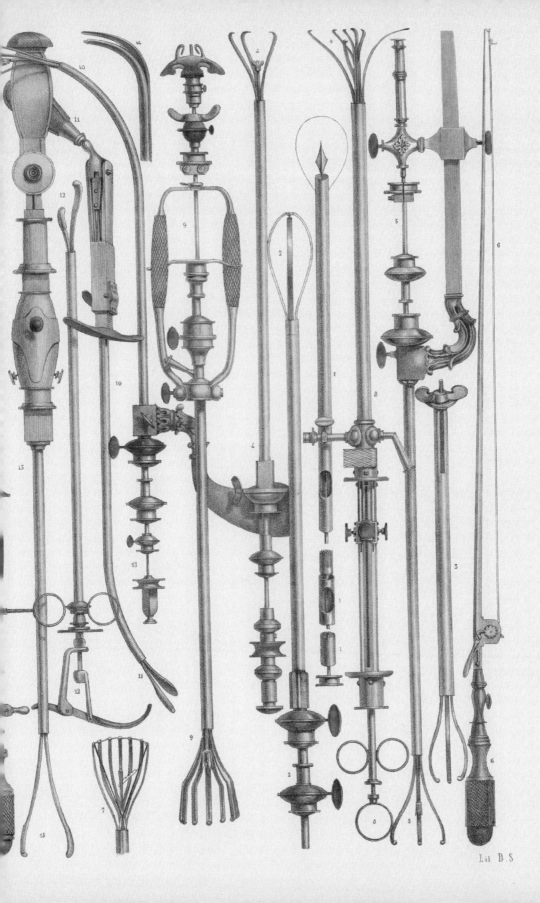

Lit. D.S

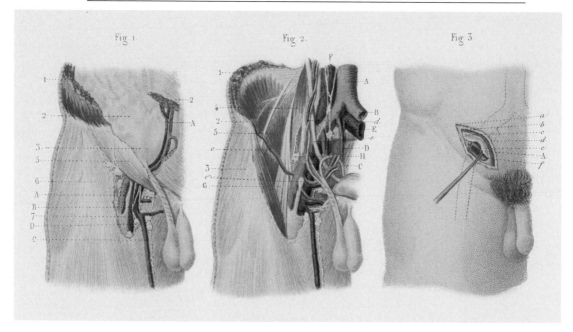

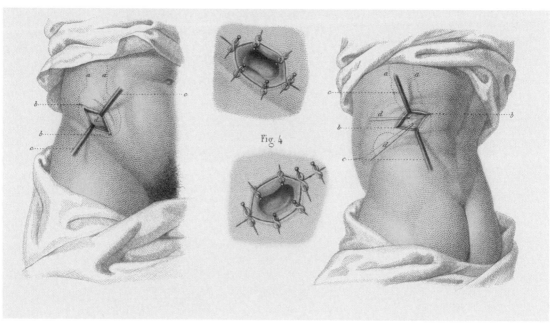

PREVIOUS: PAGE 166 | Dissection of the abdomen showing the mesentery, a membrane providing blood supply and support to the small intestine. PAGES 168-169 | Surgical instruments for lithotripsy—the breaking up and removal of kidney or bladder stones.

ABOVE: *(top)* Anatomy of the inguinal region, and ligature of the femoral, iliac and epigastric arteries. *(bottom)* Abdominal incision and opening up of the caecum (part of the large intestine).

OPPOSITE: *(top left)* Surface markers for abdominal surgery. *(top right)* Musculature and blood supply of the abdominal wall. *(bottom left)* Surgical anatomy of the large intestine (front view). *(bottom right)* Surgical anatomy of the large intestine (rear view).

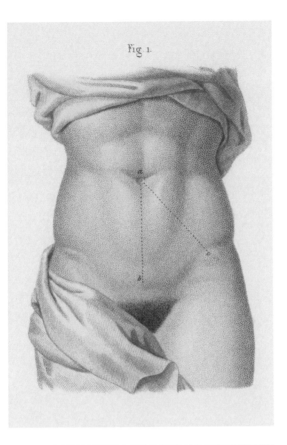

Fig. 1.

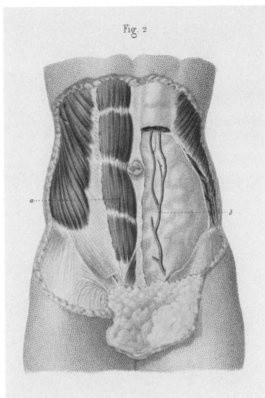

Fig. 2.

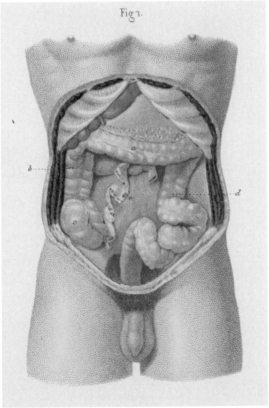

Fig. 7.

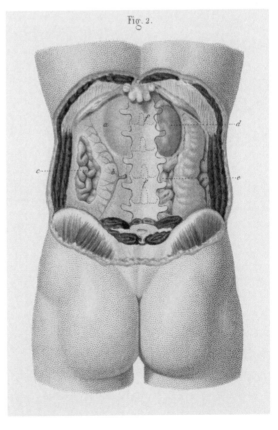

Fig. 2.

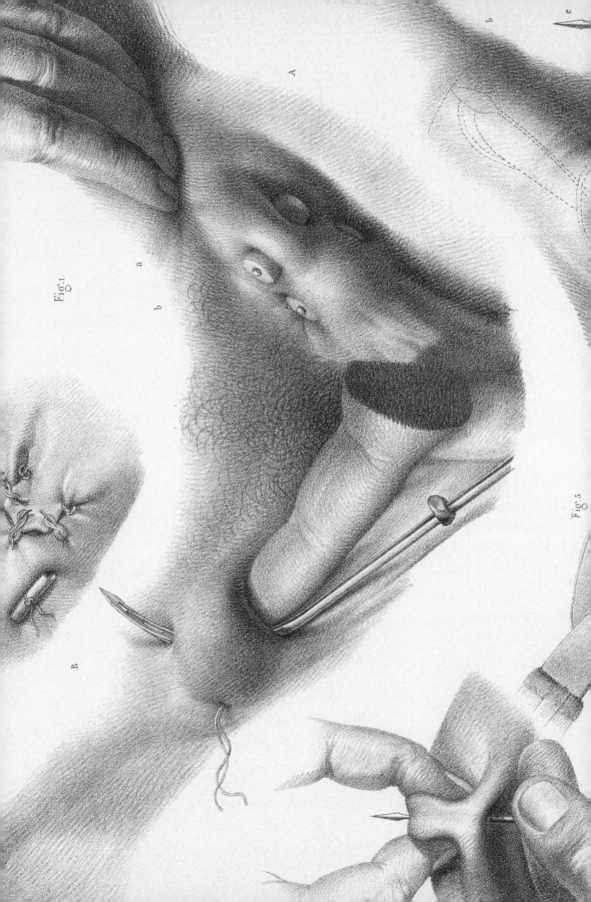

Fig.1.

a

b

A

b

e

B

Fig.5

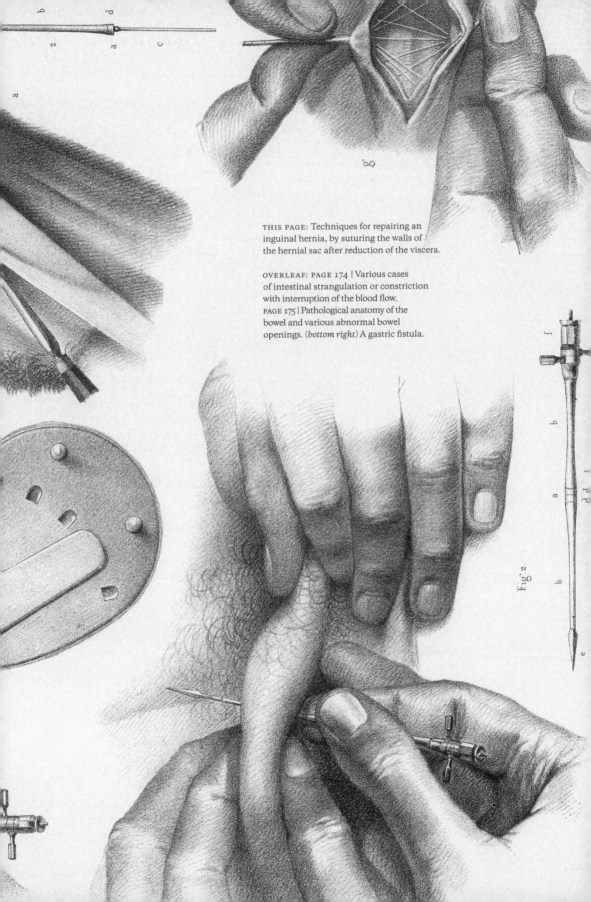

THIS PAGE: Techniques for repairing an inguinal hernia, by suturing the walls of the hernial sac after reduction of the viscera.

OVERLEAF: PAGE 174 | Various cases of intestinal strangulation or constriction with interruption of the blood flow. PAGE 175 | Pathological anatomy of the bowel and various abnormal bowel openings. (*bottom right*) A gastric fistula.

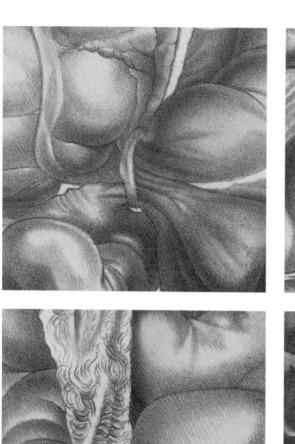
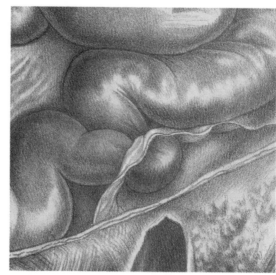
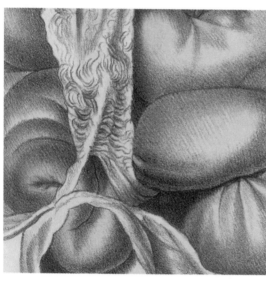
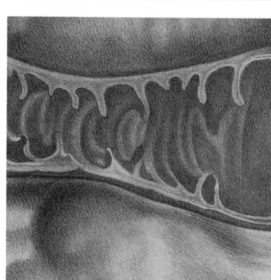
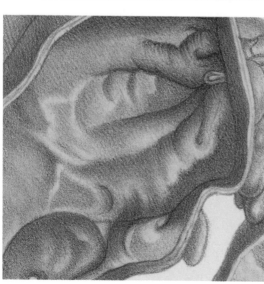
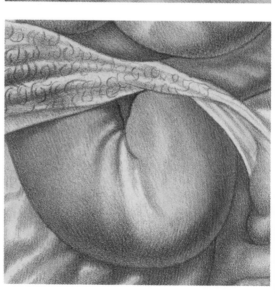

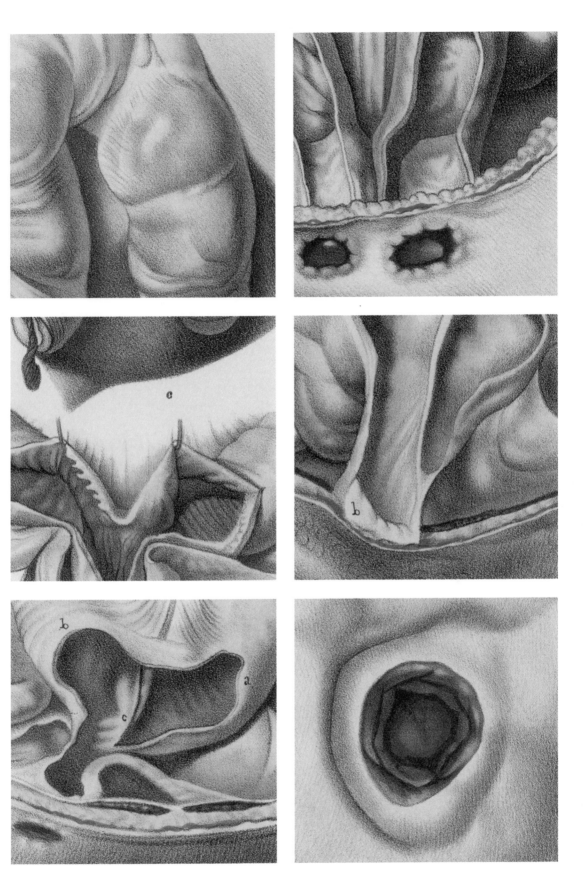

THIS PAGE: Surgical treatment of internal and external fistulas in the rectum.

OPPOSITE: Excision of haemorrhoids.

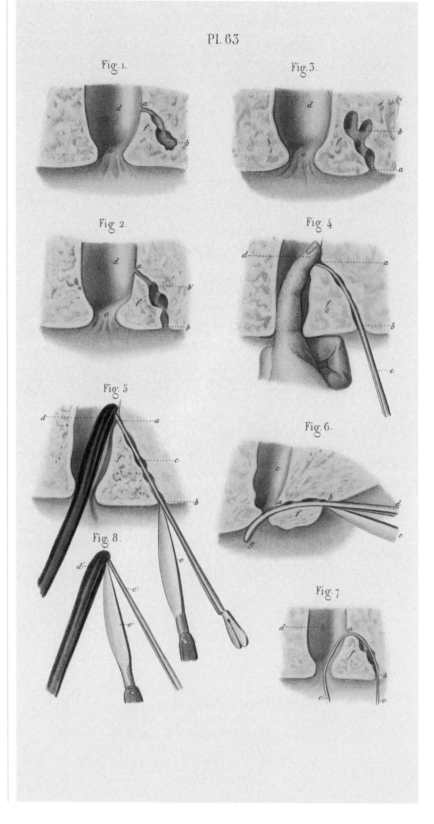

Pl. 63

Fig. 1.

Fig. 2.

Fig. 3.

Fig. 4

Fig. 5

Fig. 6.

Fig. 8.

Fig. 7

Pl. 63 bis

Fig. 1.

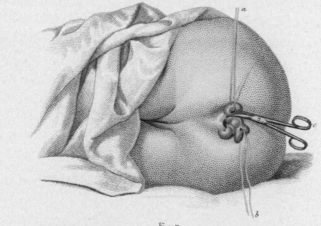

Fig. 2

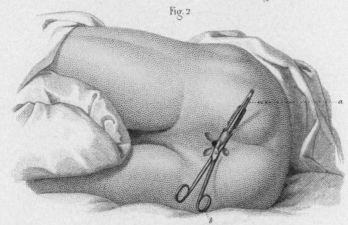

Fig 3.

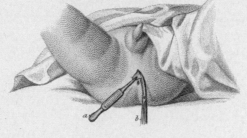

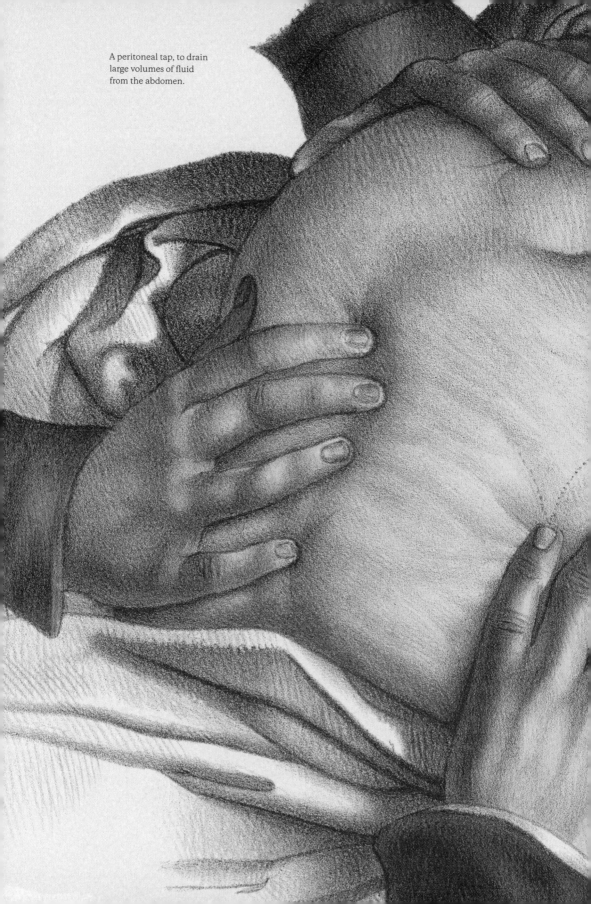

A peritoneal tap, to drain large volumes of fluid from the abdomen.

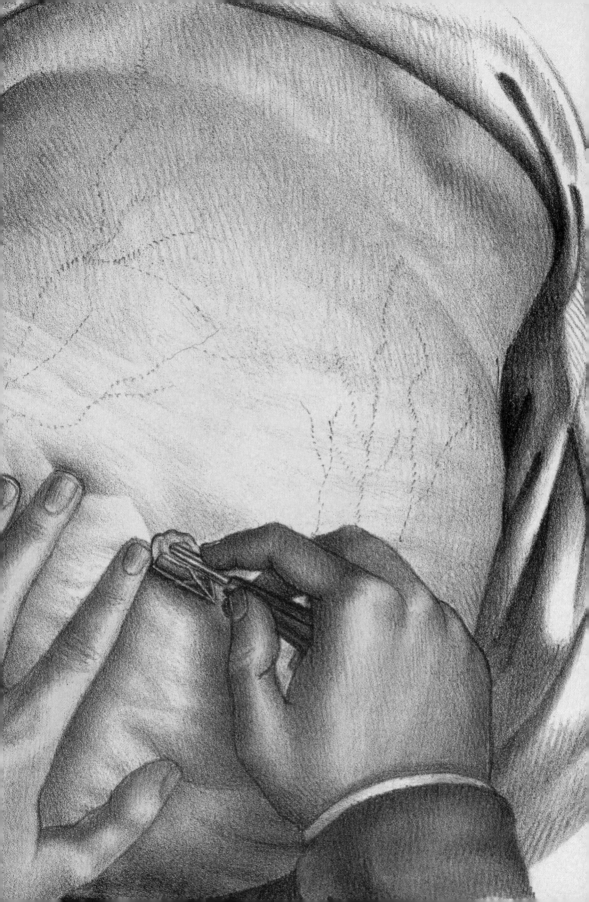

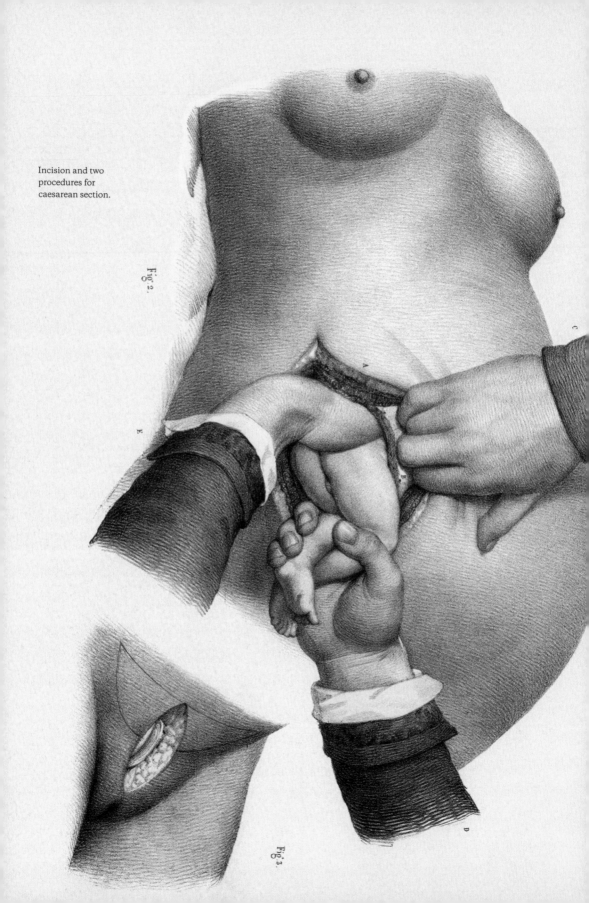

Incision and two
procedures for
caesarean section.

Fig 2.

Fig 3.

Fig. 1.

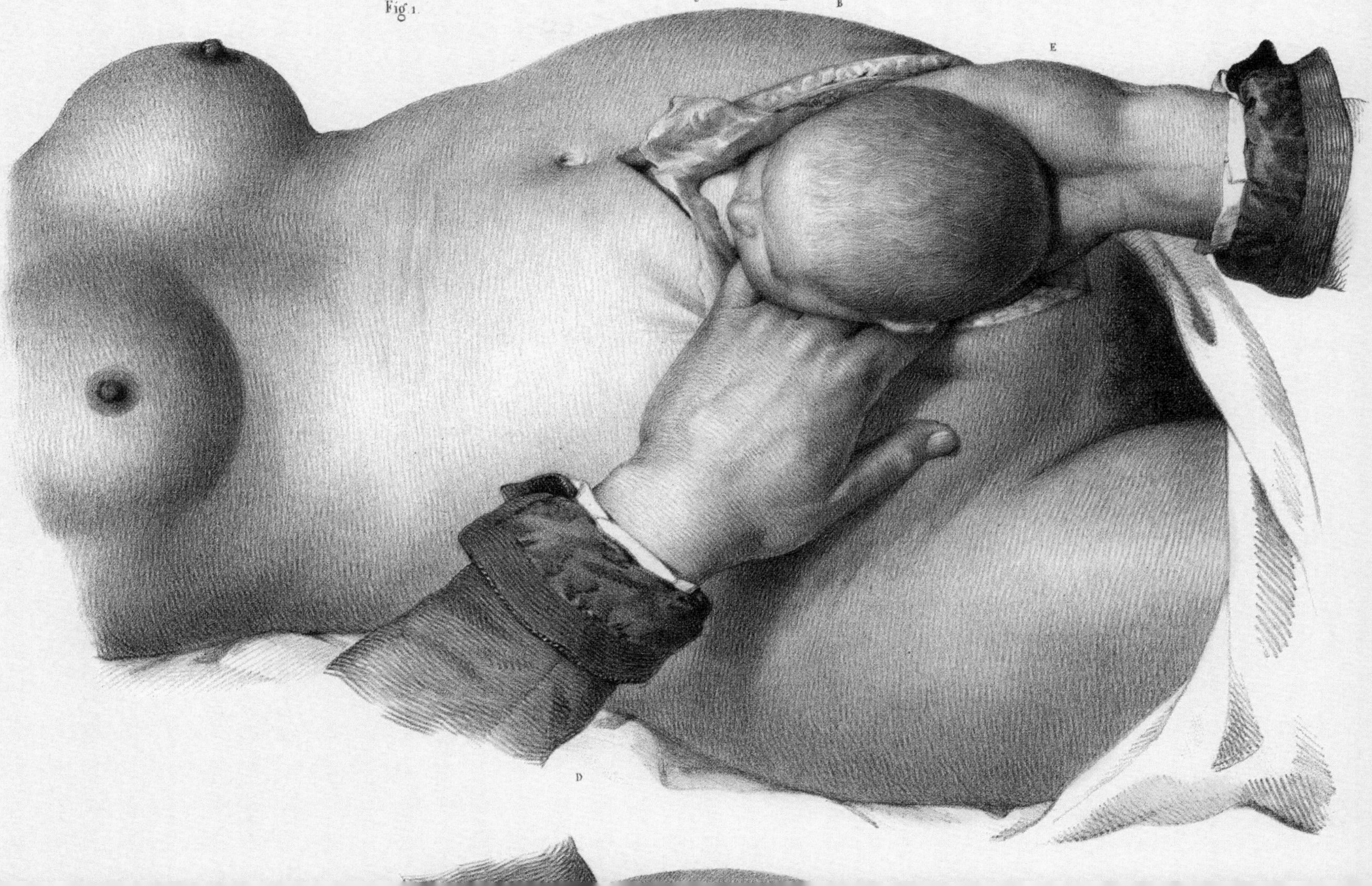

D

c
A
B

E

Pl. 77.

WALKING THE WARDS: *Teaching & Organizing Surgery.*

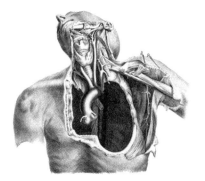

Fig. 1.

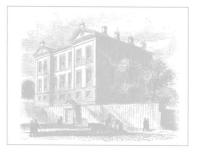

Fig. 2.

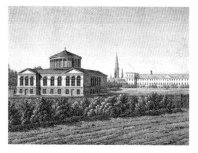

Fig. 3.

One of the themes of this book is the impact of Paris medicine—the intellectual and social transformations in medicine at the time of the French Revolution—on the development of surgery through the nineteenth century. From one perspective, this influence was practical, making localistic resection (the cutting out of diseased or damaged tissue) the main business of surgeons. But Paris medicine also changed the ways that surgeons taught their students, organized themselves as a profession, and responded to new ideas of specialist practice.

From the early nineteenth century we can begin to see the influence of Paris medicine on the teaching of surgery in Europe and the United States. American medical schools were particularly enthusiastic in adopting its precepts—one way for this young nation to distance itself from British influence after independence—and hospitals across Europe and the United States built dissecting rooms and lecture theatres to accommodate the new demand for practical teaching and observation. This new style was still controversial: George Eliot's *Middlemarch* (1871-72), set in the 1830s, shows elder medical practitioners shocked by the young Paris-trained Tertius Lydgate and his stethoscope:

> *Lydgate seemed to think the case worth a great deal of attention. He not only used his stethoscope (which had not become a matter of course in practice at that time), but sat quietly by his patient and watched him.*

Surgeons who had trained alongside physicians and saw themselves as professional equals, operating from a shared foundation of knowledge and skills, began to seek qualifications in recognition of their parity.

British governments were not yet prepared to follow the French example and establish state-funded medical schools with standardized curricula, and the task of setting and maintaining standards of surgical education fell to the new royal colleges. The Edinburgh college (chartered in 1778) and its London counterpart (chartered in 1800) both offered diplomas in surgery, and following the Apothecaries Act of 1815—the first serious British attempt to regulate clinical practice—these diplomas became entry points to British surgery. Students who had taken classes at private medical or anatomy schools and had obtained certificates of attendance, could sit for the diploma; if they succeeded, they might go on to hospital posts and, eventually, a fellowship. This system depended on trust in the quality of private surgical education, and in 1824 the London college excluded most provincial schools, on the grounds that their students were not gaining a broad experience of contemporary surgical practice. Five years later some of these schools were readmitted, on the understanding that students would spend six months walking the wards of a London teaching hospital before they could take the diploma.

At this moment of professional consolidation, Western surgery was, paradoxically, starting to fragment. Classical medicine, with its belief in diseases as a constitutional imbalance, and the genteel aspirations of its practitioners, had led physicians to see themselves as learned generalists, exponents of an art that took in every aspect of the human condition. To these clinical grandees, specialization diminished medicine: it was the sort of work suited to ignorant, narrow-minded mechanics. The anatomo-localism of Paris medicine, the idea that different tissues went

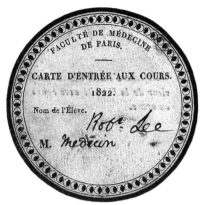

Fig. 4.

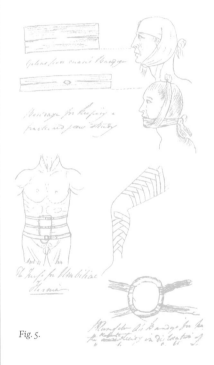

Fig. 5.

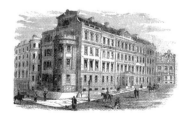

Fig. 6.

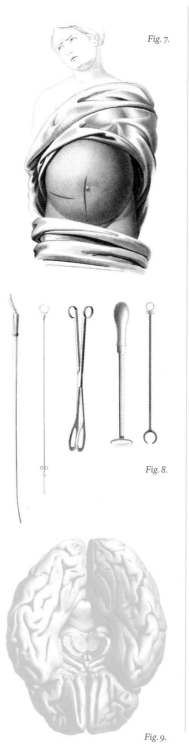

Fig. 7.

Fig. 8.

Fig. 9.

wrong in different ways, made specialization more appealing to younger practitioners, but this was not only a matter of changing clinical theories. Debates on public health sparked new concern over groups of patients or particular conditions— especially tuberculosis and venereal diseases. Large new medical schools, meanwhile, were churning out thousands of surgeons and physicians, for whom specialization was one way in which to find a profitable place in the crowded medical marketplace.

Specialization could mean many things: specialists might build their reputation around a stage of life, such as with paediatricians or obstetricians; a system of the body, such as with neurologists or orthopaedic surgeons; an organ, such as with hepatologists or eye surgeons; or a particular procedure, such as correcting stammering or squints. Staking a claim to specialist knowledge entailed publishing case reports and descriptions of techniques, and in the second half of the nineteenth century Germany was the centre of European surgical literature. The first surgical journal—the *Archiv für klinische Chirurgie*—came out in Germany in 1861, and eleven years later German surgeons created the first national surgical society. German-speaking lands also produced the first academic departments of surgery. In Berlin, Albrecht von Graefe made ophthalmic surgery into a German speciality; Emil Theodor Kocher, in Berne, used experimental thyroid physiology to develop his surgery for goitre; and, in Vienna, Theodor Billroth was the first surgeon to publish accounts of failed operations alongside his successes.

In Britain, hospitals, rather than academic departments, were the first specialist surgical institutions. By the 1860s, London was home to more than sixty specialist hospitals, from the Royal Waterloo Hospital for Children and Women and the London Cancer Hospital to the Metropolitan Ear and Throat Hospital and the Infirmary for the Relief of the Poor Afflicted with Fistula and Other Diseases of the Rectum. These places were independent charities or small businesses, and their success was a matter of supply and demand. Specialist hospitals provided security and status for ambitious young surgeons, and catered to newly prosperous members of the lower-middle classes, people who had money to spend on hospital care but could not afford the attention of what was coming to be known as Harley Street. In Britain and France surgeons preferred to publish their research and the results of their practice in the general medical press—perhaps a symbol of their greater resistance to surgical specialization—and the *British Journal of Surgery* did not appear until the eve of the First World War. Across the Atlantic, specialist hospitals in large American cities were often devoted to a particular immigrant community: Jewish, Italian, German, Irish.

By the late nineteenth century, surgical specialization was established within Western medicine, but it remained divisive. Christopher Lawrence has shown that, in this era, elite clinicians responded to the growing importance of laboratory science and complex medical equipment by emphasizing the value of broad experience and incommunicable knowledge. Thermometers and sphygmomanometers, petri dishes and microscopes were all very well, but 'only the gentleman, broadly educated, and soundly read in the classics, could be equipped for the practice of medicine'.[1] This view reflected their large and lucrative private practices, catering to patients who still expected a more Classical style of medical encounter.

Arguments over incommunicable knowledge were, of course, hardly new to surgeons, who had suffered the disdain of learned physicians for centuries, and their practice had always involved specialist instruments. Equally, elite surgeons could argue that their practice, not that of physicians, was the exemplum of incommunicable knowledge. Laboratory specialists were beginning to take a role

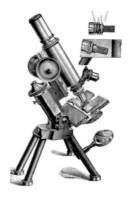

Fig. 10.

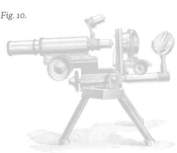

Fig. 11.

[1] Christopher Lawrence, 'Incommunicable knowledge: science, technology and the clinical art in Britain, 1850–1914', *Journal of Contemporary History* 20, 1985.

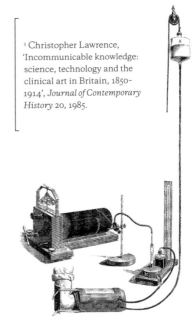

Fig. 12.

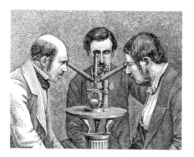

Fig. 13.

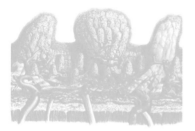

Fig. 14.

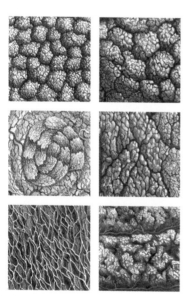

Fig. 15.

in the surgical diagnosis of diseases such as cancer. The naked-eye 'clinical gaze' of Paris medicine had its limits, and by the end of the nineteenth century surgeons were sending pieces of excised tissue to laboratory pathologists. These specialists could, with the aid of a microscope, distinguish tumours from syphilitic or tuberculous growths, and—crucially—give some sense of whether a cancer might be malignant. New laboratory equipment such as the freezing microtome allowed these histological diagnoses to be done quickly, in some cases while the patient was still anaesthetized and on the operating table. Surgeons continued to insist upon the final word, and sometimes criticized pathologists for their vague or non-committal diagnoses. But in this way, surgeons and scientists collaborated in determining the course of treatment and its urgency, a form of shared expertise that would become central to surgery in the twentieth century and beyond. What we think of as modern surgery—surgeons and their juniors, anaesthetists, theatre nurses, specialists in imaging technologies such as MRI, intensive care physicians and so on—is a fundamentally collaborative business, relying on the interplay between myriad forms of specialist expertise.

At the end of the nineteenth century, surgeons had adopted the traditional hallmarks of medical practice, and leading surgeons prided themselves on their hospital appointments and their large private practices. But at the very moment that this new surgical circle proclaimed the triumph of scientific surgery, it was also resisting the encroachment of laboratory science on its authority. Surgery might be scientific, but it was also—using language going back centuries—an art, and a matter of clinical judgement developed over a lifetime, rather than a basic skill that could be mass-produced in medical schools or laboratories.

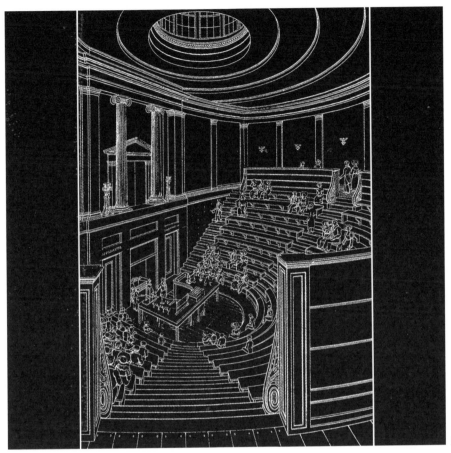

Fig. 16.

FIG. 1: *No matter how crisp and detailed anatomical illustration became—and this engraving by Joseph Maclise (1815-1880) is remarkable—surgical skill could never be acquired from texts and images alone.* FIG. 2: *Within a generation, the Paris style of clinical teaching was in use at American medical schools such as the New York Medical College.* FIG. 3: *New medical schools, such as this one in Bonn, borrowed the Parisian idea of surgical education through dissection and practical experience on the wards.* FIG. 4: *Despite the Napoleonic Wars (1799-1815) and their long aftermath, students came from across Europe and the United States to study medicine and surgery in Paris.* FIG. 5: *These notes, made by one D. D. Dobree during lectures by the surgeon John Abernethy (1764-1831) in 1814, give us some idea of what techniques surgical students were expected to learn.* FIG. 6: *Students at Charing Cross Hospital Medical School—one of the largest in London—faced the problem of an increasingly crowded medical marketplace.* FIG. 7: *Well before the advent of anaesthesia in 1846, surgeons were being taught complex abdominal operations such as caesarean section.* FIG. 8: *From the middle of the eighteenth century, 'man-midwives' or* accoucheurs *began to encroach on the traditionally female territory of supervising childbirth.* FIG. 9: *Learning anatomy by dissection brought surgical and medical students together to think about the fine structure and function of the body.* FIG. 10: *Microscopes such as these extended the 'clinical gaze' of Paris medicine to the body's tissues and cells.* FIG. 11: *Inexpensive teaching microscopes became a common feature of medical and surgical classrooms in the late nineteenth century.* FIG. 12: *While Paris medicine focused on anatomy, the new discipline of physiology began to study bodily function with instruments such as the sphygmomanometer.* FIG. 13: *How to make sure that students saw the same things down their microscopes? This three-barrelled French microscope offered one solution.* FIG. 14: *Specialization led surgeons and physicians to take an even closer interest in the fine structure of tissues such as the skin.* FIG. 15: *In a culture obsessed with appearance and cleanliness, dermatology could be a profitable speciality.* FIG. 16: *As surgery embraced the rhetoric of science, its architecture—such as the lecture theatre of the London Institution—continued to proclaim a connection with Classical learning.*

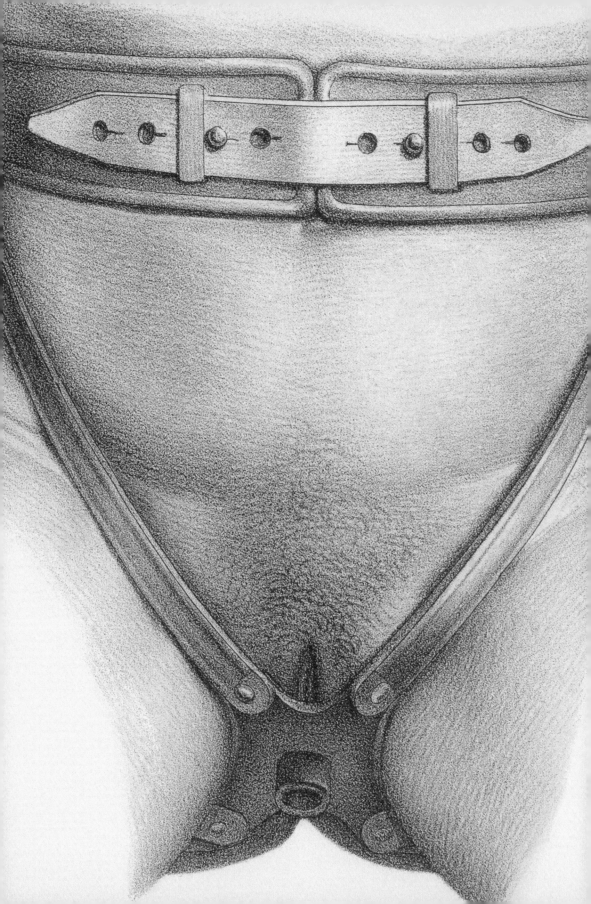

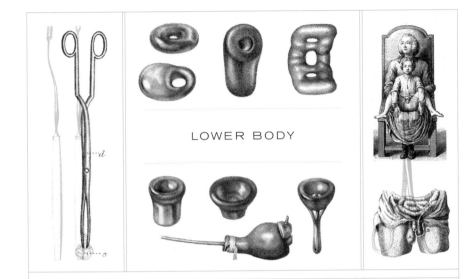

LOWER BODY

GENITALS.

VII

189

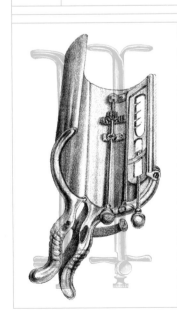

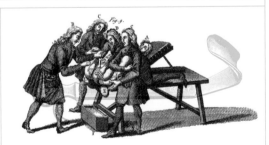

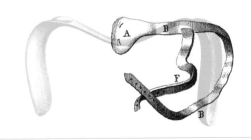

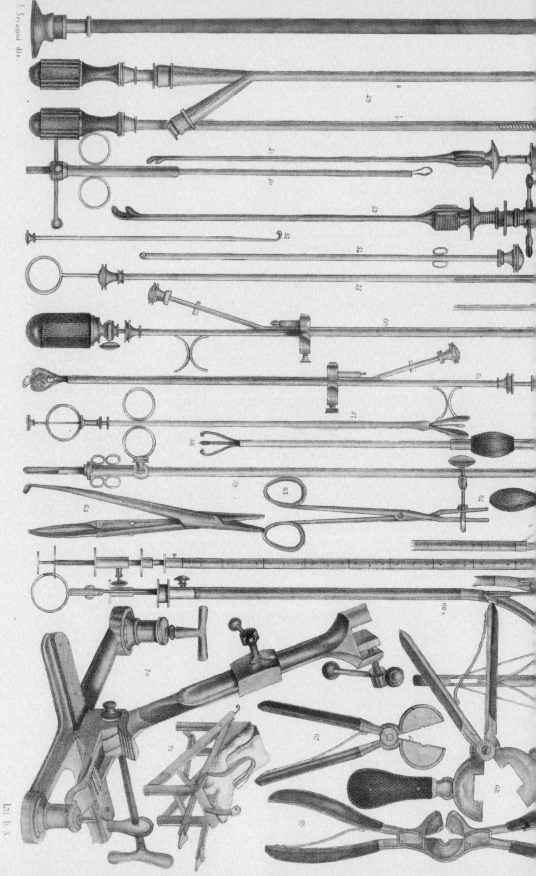

Serafini dis.

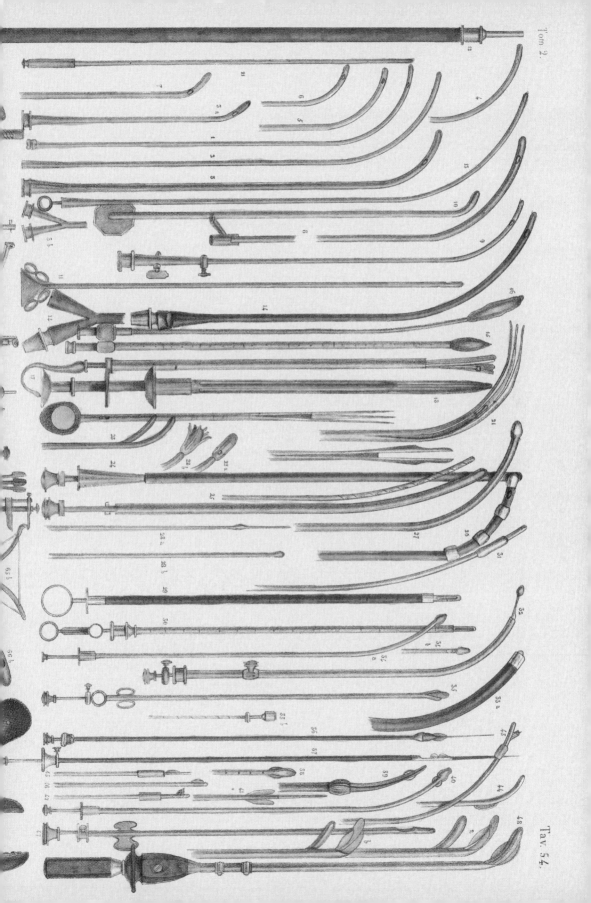

Pl. 67.

Fig   Fig.   Fig

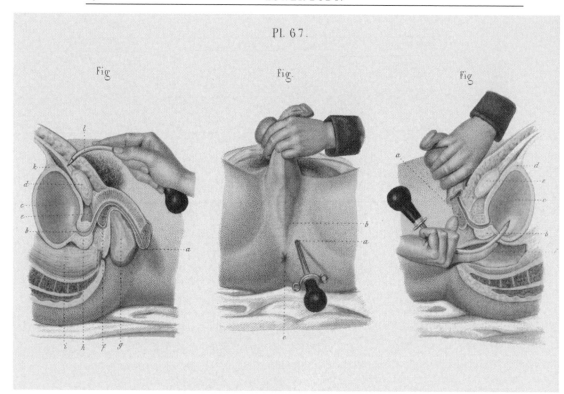

Pl. 68

Fig 1   Fig. 2.

Fig. 3.   Fig. 4

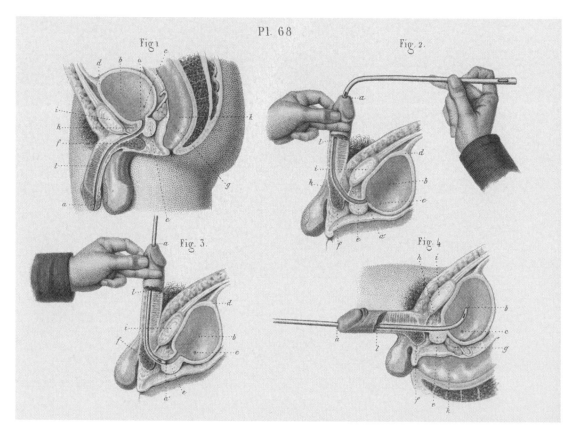

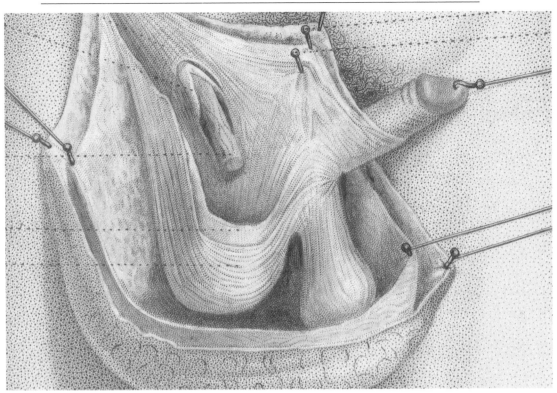

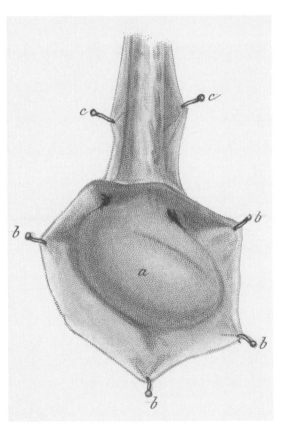

PREVIOUS: PAGE 188 | Treatment of a prolapsed uterus, with a pessary held in position by an abdominal belt and straps. PAGES 190–191 | Surgical instruments and catheters for operating on the male genito-urinary system.

OPPOSITE: *(top)* Surgical puncture of the bladder. *(bottom)* Insertion of a surgical catheter in a male patient.

THIS PAGE: *(top)* Surgical anatomy of the inguinal canal and scrotum. *(bottom)* Surgical anatomy of the testis and spermatic cord.

OVERLEAF: *(left)* Surgical procedure for relieving phimosis (tight foreskin) and paraphimosis (trapping of the foreskin behind the head of the penis). *(right)* Illustrations of urethral stricture and its surgical relief via urethroplasty.

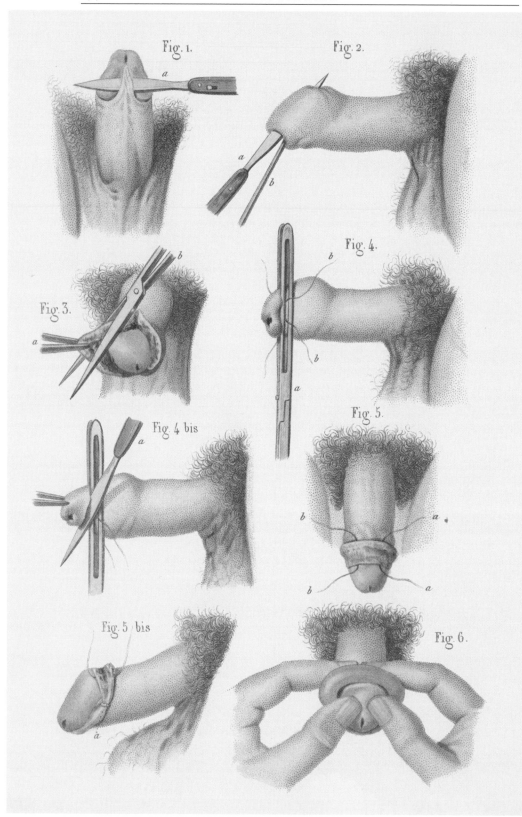

Fig. 1.

Fig. 2.

Fig. 3.

Fig. 4.

Fig. 4 bis

Fig. 5.

Fig. 5 bis

Fig. 6.

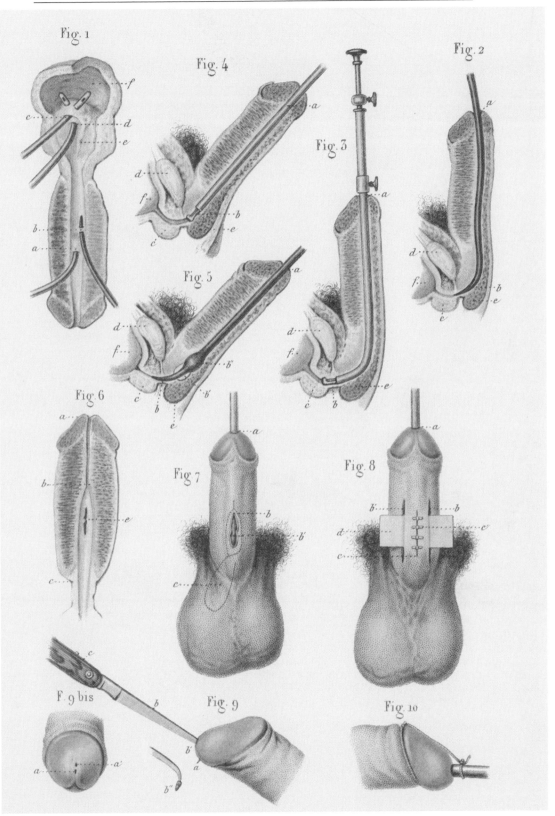

Fig. 1
Fig. 4
Fig. 2
Fig. 3
Fig. 5
Fig. 6
Fig. 7
Fig. 8
F. 9 bis
Fig. 9
Fig. 10

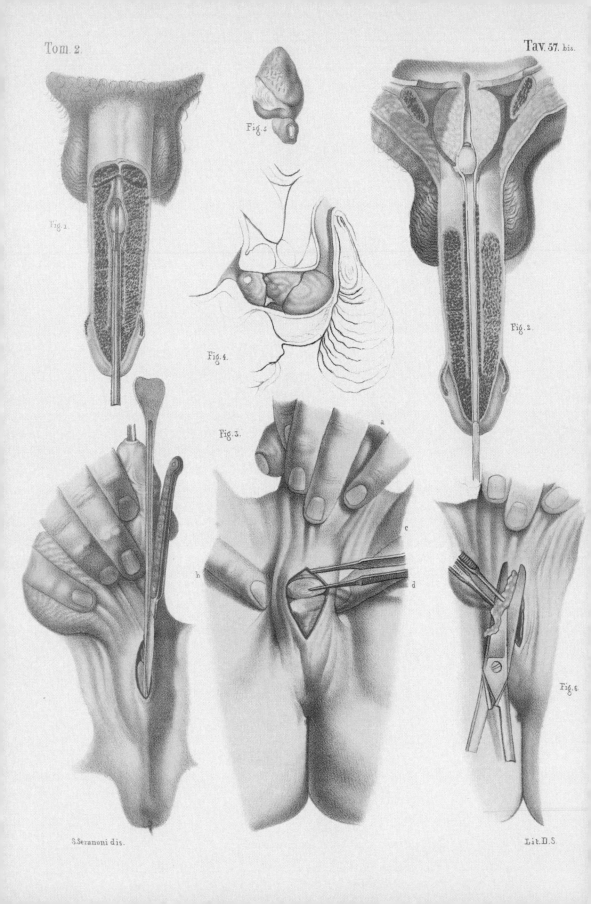

Fig. 5.

Fig. 1.

Fig. 2.

Fig. 4.

Fig. 3.

Fig. 6.

S. Seranoni dis.

Lit. D.S.

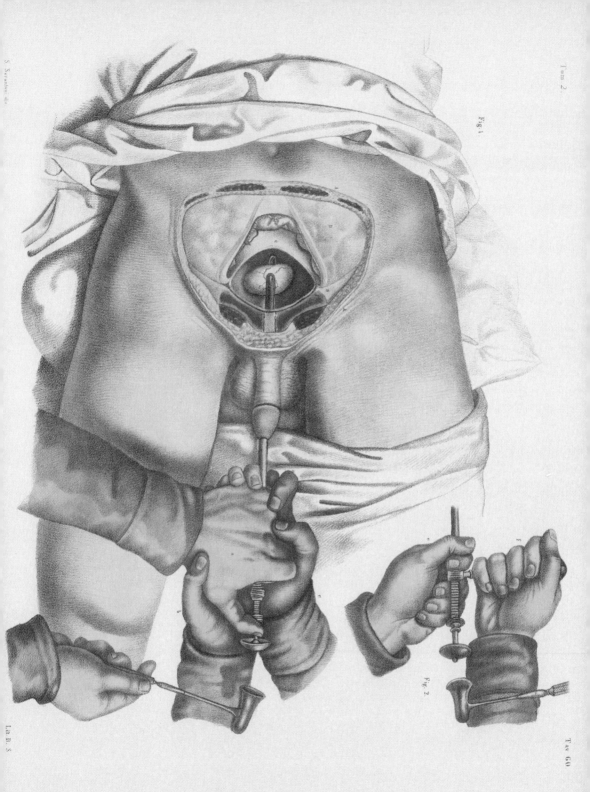

Fig. 2.

Ln B. S

Tav 60

OPPOSITE: Procedure for the removal of stones from the prostate, urethra and penis.
ABOVE: The use of a catheter, clamp and hammer to shatter bladder stones *in situ*.

THIS PAGE:
Surgical removal of
testicular tumours,
and amputation of
the head of the penis.

OPPOSITE:
Surgical treatment
of a varicocele
(a mass of enlarged
veins in the testis).

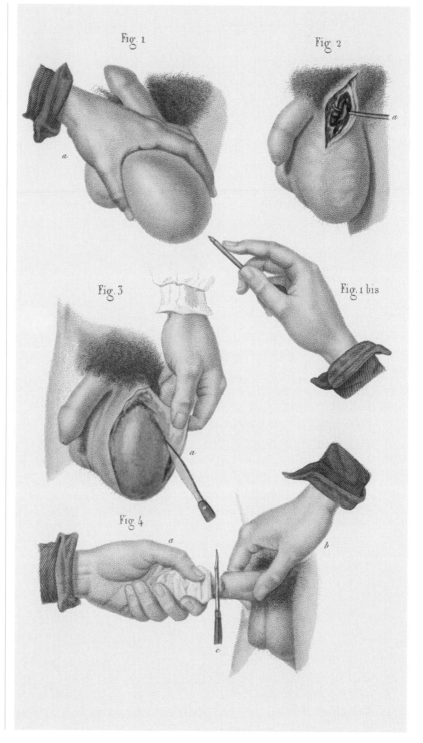

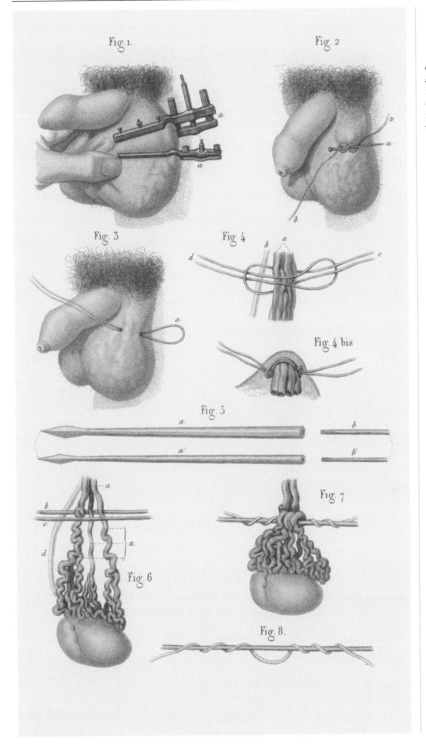

Fig. 1.

Fig. 2

Fig. 3

Fig. 4

Fig. 4 bis

Fig. 5

Fig. 6

Fig. 7

Fig. 8.

OVERLEAF:
A selection of
instruments for
operating on the
female genitals,
vagina and uterus.

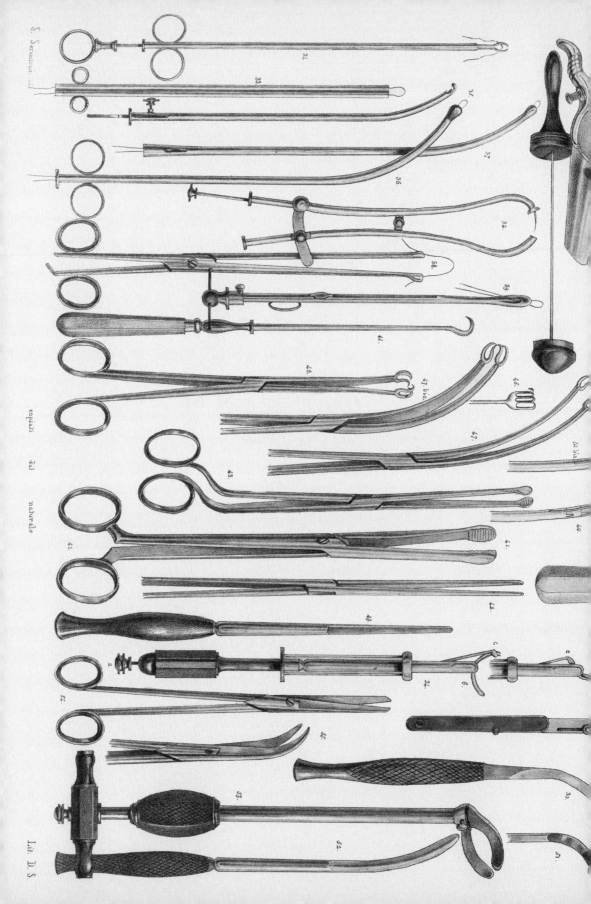

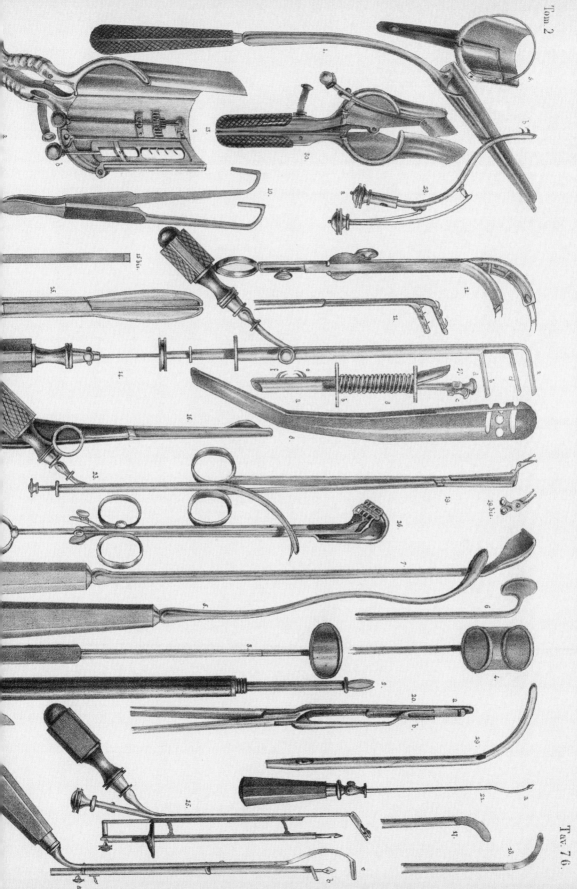

The musculature and veins of the female pelvis and genitals.

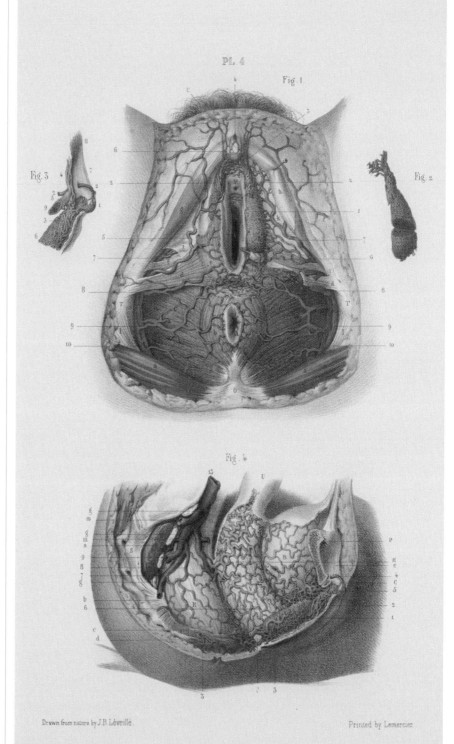

Drawn from nature by J.B. Léveillé.

Printed by Lemercier.

The anatomy of the
female pelvic floor, vagina,
uterus and ovaries.

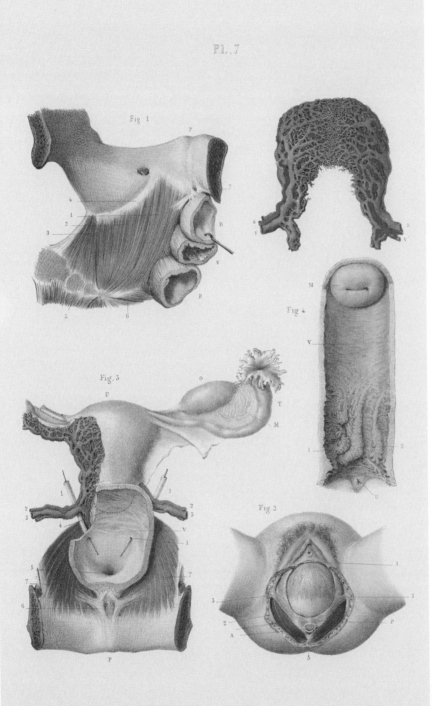

PL. 7

Fig 1

Fig. 3

Fig 4

Fig 2

Drawn by J B Léveillé

Printed by Lemercier Paris

Instruments and techniques for surgery of the cervix and uterus.

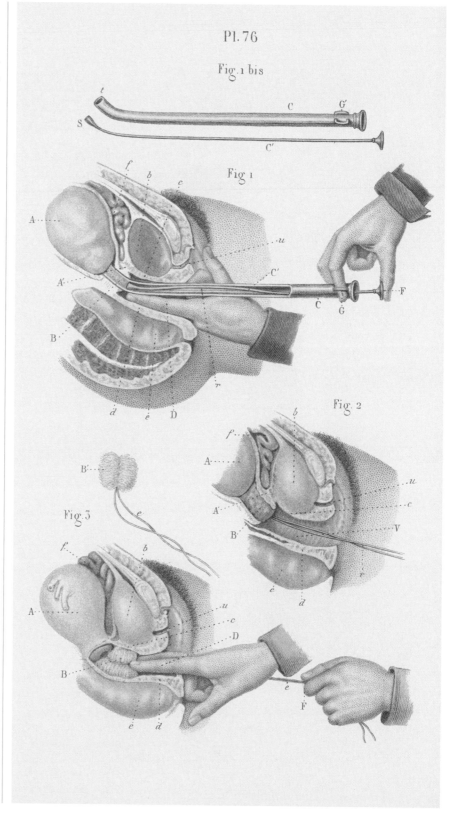

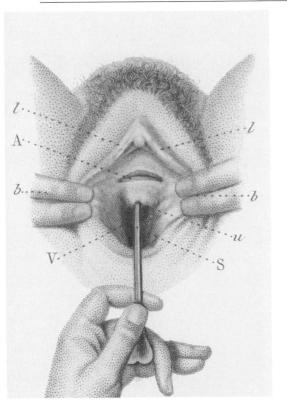

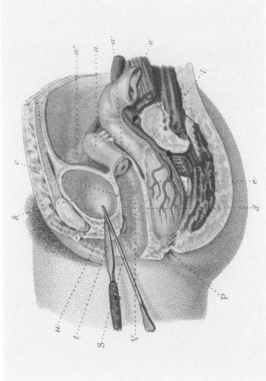

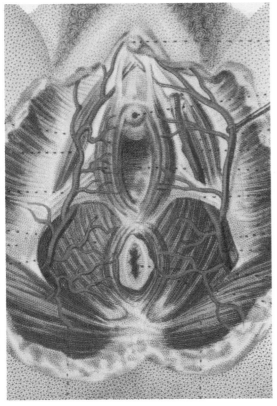

THIS PAGE: *(top left)* The anatomy of the female external and internal genitals. *(top right)* The anatomy of the female pelvis. *(left)* The musculature of the female pelvic floor.

OVERLEAF: PAGE 206 *(top left)* Suturing of an incision in the female perineum. *(top right)* The lymphatic drainage of the female pelvis and genital organs. *(bottom left)* The anatomy and venous drainage of the female pelvis. *(bottom right)* The anatomy of the uterus. PAGE 207 *(top left)* Surgical repair of damage to the perineum. *(top right)* The lymphatic and venous drainage of the female inguinal canal. *(bottom left)* The lymphatic drainage of the female pelvis. *(bottom right)* The anatomy of the female external and internal genitals.

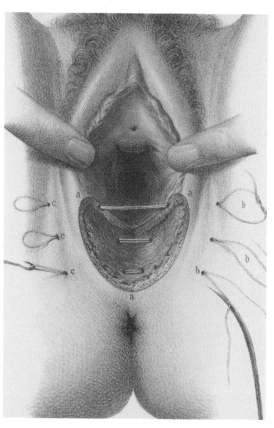

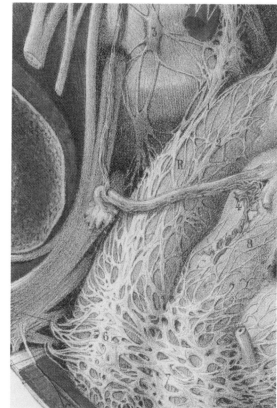

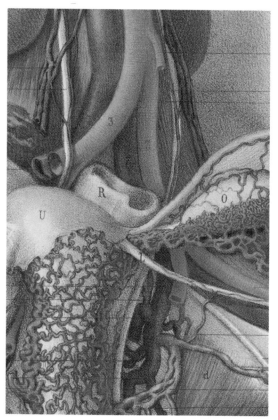

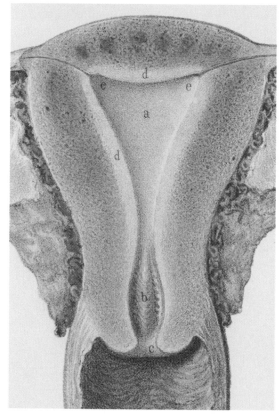

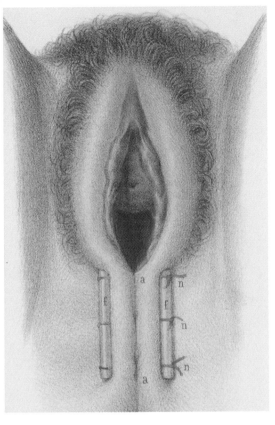

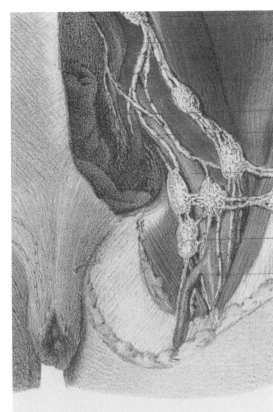

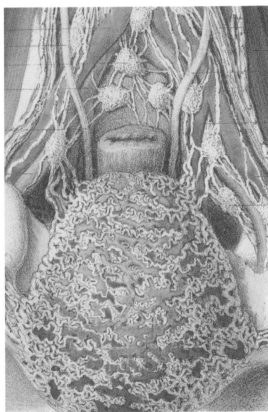

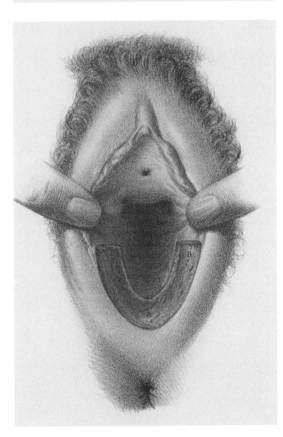

THIS PAGE: Surgical procedures for removing uterine polyps and repairing a prolapsed uterus.

OPPOSITE: Surgical procedure for the repair of a vesico-vaginal fistula.

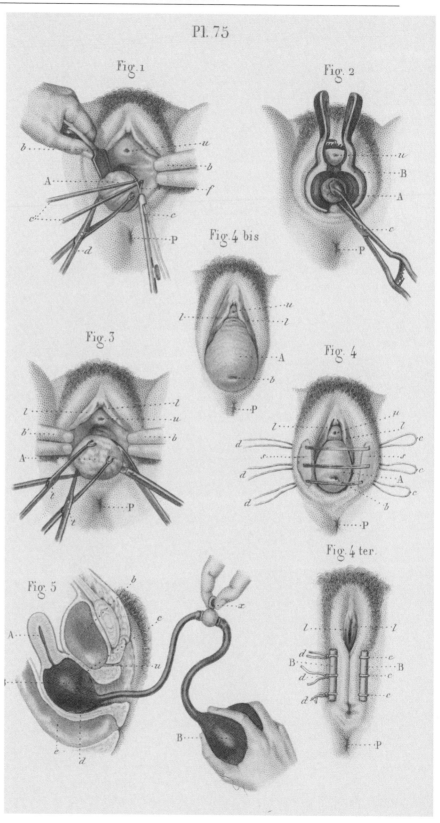

Pl. 75

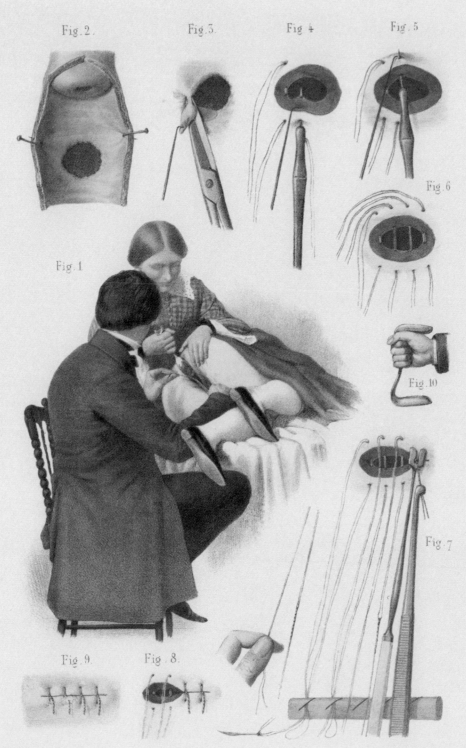

SO SIMPLE & SO GRAND: *Surgery in 1900.*

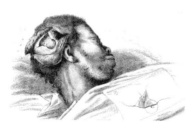

Fig. 1.

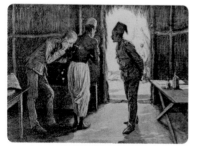

Fig. 2.

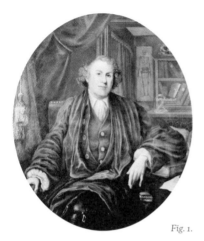

Fig. 3.

How would surgeons have described themselves
and their practice at the turn of the twentieth
century? Heroic, humane, scientific, experimental,
unselfish, democratic, near-divine—all these words
can be found in contemporary descriptions of
surgery by surgeons. Addressing the International
Congress of Arts and Science in 1904, the American
surgeon Frederick Dennis went even further:

*The science of surgery stands out in bold relief, and
conspicuous grandeur, apart from and above the
others, in that it deals directly with human life, that
most precious of mortal possessions, often lending to
it not only a helping, but a saving hand. At the same
time, its story is so simple and so grand, that the child
and the savant may alike participate in the pleasure
which the wonderful narrative is fitted to convey.*

This story of hard-won surgical progress was
reshaped radically, according to the purposes
for which it was being told. In Britain, alongside
engineering and exploration, surgery was claimed
as the outstanding achievement of imperial
civilization—and a justification of the global
reach of the British Empire. In the United States,
by contrast, surgeons were portrayed as pioneers,
embodiments of the frontier spirit. As Dennis wrote:

*There is no science that calls for greater fearlessness,
courage and nerve than that of surgery, none*

*that demands more of self-reliance, principle,
independence and the determination in the man.*

Looking beyond their particular national
perspectives, surgeons across Europe and the
United States could at last agree that their profession
was technically assured and secure, beyond question.
Textbooks, such as Emil Theodor Kocher's
Chirurgische Operationslehre (1907), showed that
there was no part of the body on which surgeons did
not operate. Although the Nobel Prizes, instituted
in 1901, had no separate category for surgery, within
a decade two surgeons—Kocher, for his work on
the thyroid, and the French surgeon Alexis Carrel,
for his innovations in suturing blood vessels—had
received the prize in physiology or medicine. A
generation of surgeons—Joseph Lister in Britain,
Harvey Cushing in the US, Theodor Billroth in
Germany—were acclaimed as national heroes
and 'fathers' of their respective surgical traditions,
for which they were well-rewarded, earning more
than the leaders of the medical profession.

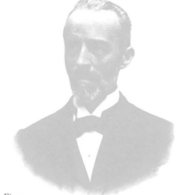

Fig. 4.

However, these surgeons were beginning to
grapple with practical challenges that could not
be answered with operative skill and anatomical
expertise. For those experimenting with tissue
transplants between patients, why did the
overwhelming majority of these operations fail?
If damaged joints were to be replaced, not just
removed, what materials would be most suitable?
And if surgery was to be a tool of diagnosis as well
as treatment, how could its practitioners examine
the interior of their patients' bodies while causing
as little damage as possible? As surgeons looked
ahead to new directions in surgical research, they
also looked back in new ways, revising historical
foundations for the notion of scientific surgery.

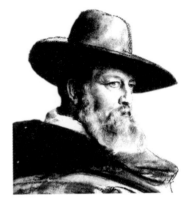

Fig. 5.

The reputation of the Scottish surgeon John
Hunter in the century after his death in 1793
reveals a great deal about the relationship between
surgery's past and its aspirations for the future.
Though his first biographer, the surgeon Jesse Foot,

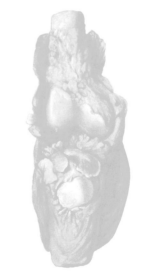

Fig. 6.

[1] L. S. Jacyna, 'Images of John Hunter in the nineteenth century', *History of Science*, 1983,

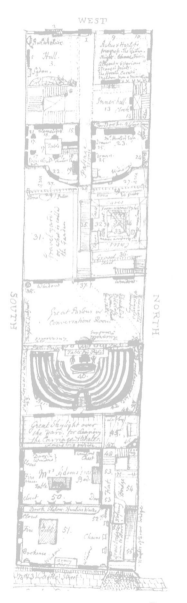

Fig. 7.

took a harder line, by the 1820s Hunter's former colleagues and students were praising him to the point of mythology as the founder of scientific surgery, and this continued into the twentieth century. As Stephen Jacyna has argued, this was not because Hunter's formidable and polymathic body of work had actually revolutionized the clinical practice of surgery.[1] Hunter was taken up because of what he represented—or, to put it more precisely, what he could be made to represent.

From 1813, Hunter's executors endowed an annual Hunterian Oration at the Royal College of Surgeons of London, to pay, in their orotund words:

… a tribute of praise to those Practitioners in Surgery, who when alive contributed by their labours to the advancement of that profession which we are now anxious still further to improve.

The purpose of the Oration was to forge a clear and direct link between surgery's past and its future; stories of glorious founding fathers, such as Hunter, surely would spur modern surgeons to ever greater achievement. Looking back over their own century, late nineteenth-century surgeons identified two central episodes in surgical history. While their predecessors had framed Enlightenment surgery as a golden age of rationality after the crude ignorance of medieval practice, they saw the eighteenth century as the 'age of agony', brought to an end only with the emergence of anaesthesia and aseptic surgery—both, they thought, products of the tradition established by Hunter. In his 1877 Hunterian Oration—described in the *British Journal of Psychiatry* as 'neat and graceful, but not very deeply thought out'—the English surgeon James Paget made explicit the link between social and intellectual progress. Hunter, Paget said, 'did more than anyone to make us gentlemen', but he must also be recognized as 'the founder of scientific surgery'.

One case at the beginning of the twentieth century captures the new power and status of scientific surgery. A few days before his coronation, Edward VII—whose appetite had gained him the nickname 'Prince of Whales'—began to complain of abdominal pain. The aged Lister was called in, and recommended an operation to drain an abscess on his appendix. Carried out on 24 June 1902 by Frederick Treves, the king's Serjeant-Surgeon, the surgery was a complete success. Edward was crowned a month later, and Treves received a baronetcy. Surgeons, not physicians, had been called in to treat the highest in the land, the surgery had been carried out in accordance with current scientific thinking, the abdomen had been opened up and closed safely, and a condition that even a generation earlier might have proved fatal was resolved with a quick and simple operation.

The development of the appendectomy itself shows the growing confidence of surgeons in overturning the conventional practices and treatments established by physicians. Until the 1890s the standard response to severe abdominal pain was conservative: relieve the pain with opiates, and wait. Sir William Osler, a Canadian physician and one of the founders of Johns Hopkins Hospital, captured this view with characteristic diplomacy in his *Principles and Practice of Medicine*, published in 1892. Though he acknowledged that 'perforating appendicitis is in more than three fourths of all cases a surgical affection', he also argued that surgical intervention should always be subordinate to the authority of a physician:

> *Post mortem examinations show that the appendix is very frequently the seat of extensive disease, past or present, without the symptoms pointing to trouble.... If we regard every case of inflammation in the caecal region as appendicitis, a large proportion of the cases recover.... Post mortem observations show that very many instances get well, often without treatment.*

At the same time, however, surgeons were beginning to assert their own views on the matter.

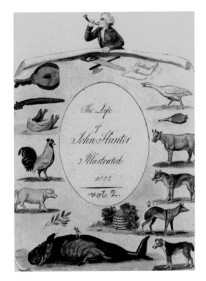

Fig. 8.

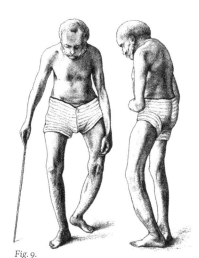

Fig. 9.

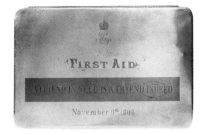

Fig. 10.

In a long essay in the *Transactions of the American Surgical Association*, published the following year, the American surgeon John Deaver made a compelling humanitarian case for early surgical intervention:

> The treatment which to my mind offers the best opportunity for permanent relief is that of immediate removal of the offending appendix as soon as the diagnosis is established. My reason for adopting such a radical course has been forced upon me by the large number of cases I have seen perish when well-directed medical means had failed to afford relief.

Deaver's colleague Richard A. Harte put it more bluntly—'Conservatism in appendicitis is a great mistake'—and within a generation this view prevailed: appendectomies were commonplace operations, straightforward and even rather dull.

Another story, in a less exalted setting, casts a different light on the state of surgery to come. Hugh Owen Thomas and his nephew Robert Jones—respectively a GP and a surgeon working in Liverpool at the turn of the century—were trained in scientific surgery and applied aseptic practice, but they also drew on a long family tradition of bonesetting, using techniques handed down over more than a century. Thomas drew on this tradition to invent the Thomas splint, a way of immobilizing broken legs that saved thousands of lives in the First World War and won him an international reputation, while Jones developed his family's insight into orthopaedic surgery and reorganized British orthopaedics during the war. Their work shows that, even at the apex of surgical achievement and ambition, we still find fruitful connections between the craft tradition and surgical modernity.

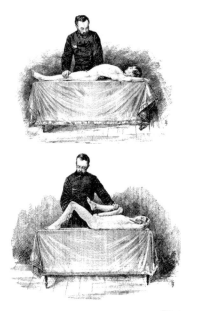

Fig. 11.

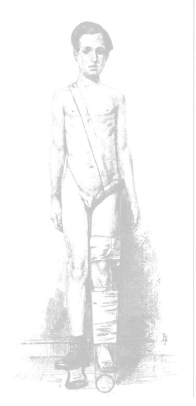

Fig. 12.

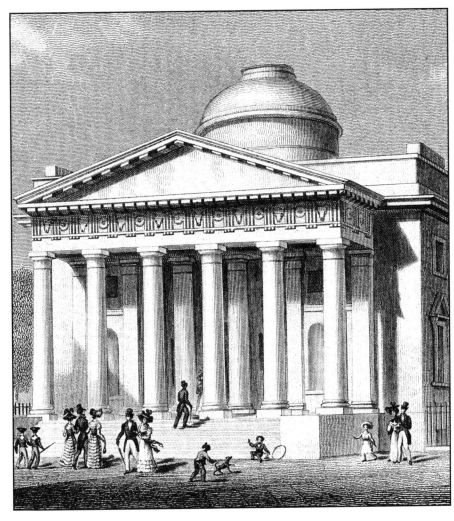

Fig. 13.

FIG. 1: *An icon of surgical enlightenment: portrait of the surgeon John Hunter (1728-1793), after Joshua Reynolds.*
FIG. 2: *By the end of the nineteenth century, no part of the human body—even the brain, as shown here—was without a surgical speciality.* FIG. 3: *Some British writers presented surgery as an outstanding achievement of Imperial civilization—and hence a humanitarian justification for British colonial rule.* FIG. 4: *The Swiss surgeon Emil Theodor Kocher (1841-1917), winner of the 1909 Nobel Prize in Physiology or Medicine.* FIG. 5: *Theodor Billroth (1829-1894), professor of surgery at the University of Vienna.* FIG. 6: *Could surgeons find new ways to treat conditions such as tubercular synovitis without merely amputating the affected joint?* FIG. 7: *A surgical polymath at work and play: this drawing of John Hunter's house and anatomy school on Leicester Square dates from 1832.* FIG. 8: *Hunter's surgical interests went beyond the merely human, and his anatomical collection included many of the creatures shown on the title page of Jesse Foot's 1822 biography.* FIG. 9: *Sir James Paget (1814-1899) was a gifted surgeon, and also identified the bone disease, shown here, that bears his name.* FIG. 10: *From November 1904, the accident-prone King Edward VII (1841-1910) carried this first-aid kit in his car.* FIG. 11: *The Welsh GP and surgeon Hugh Owen Thomas (1834-1891) drew on scientific surgery and his family's tradition of bonesetting to develop a new method for treating bone deformities.*
FIG. 12: *Thomas' simple hip splint, shown here, was intended to correct deformities of the leg.* FIG. 13: *The Hunter brothers' name is still part of the British cultural landscape: William (1718-1783) has a museum named after him in Glasgow (shown here), and John (1728-1793) in London.*

Pl. 2.

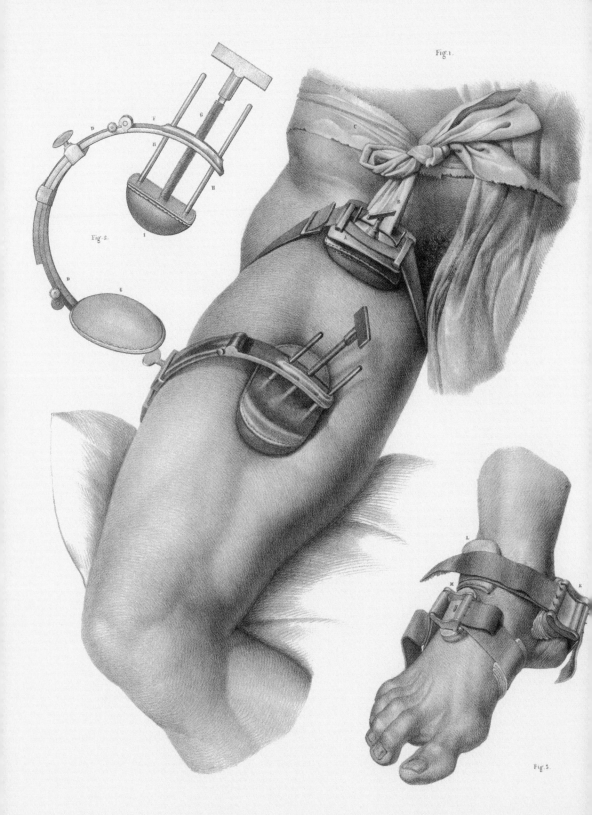

Fig. 1.

Fig. 2.

Fig. 3.

Dessiné d'après nature par N.H. Jacob.

Instrument de la Fabrique de Mr Charrière.

Lith. de Lemercier, Benard

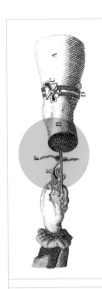

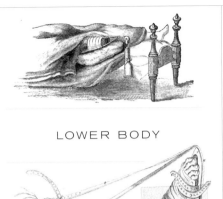

LOWER BODY

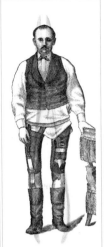

VIII

LEGS & FEET.

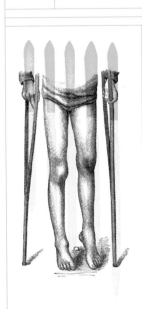

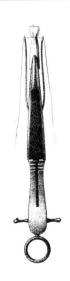

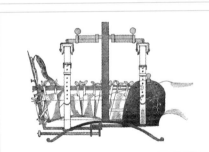

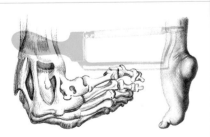

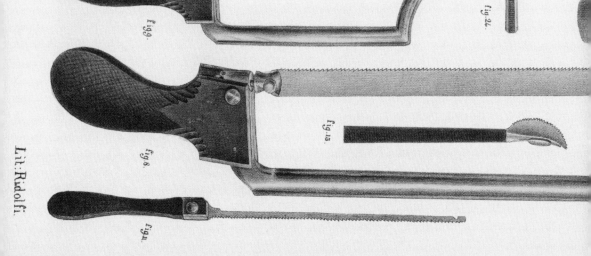

Ott: Muzzi dis.

Istrumenti fabbricati dal Sr. Charrière.

Lit: Ridolfi.

f. 1.

f. 2.

f. 3.

f. 4.

f. 5.

f. 6.

f. 7.

fig. 10.

fig. 12.

fig. 9.

fig. 8.

fig. 11.

fig. 13.

fig. 25.

fig. 26.

fig. 27.

fig. 24.

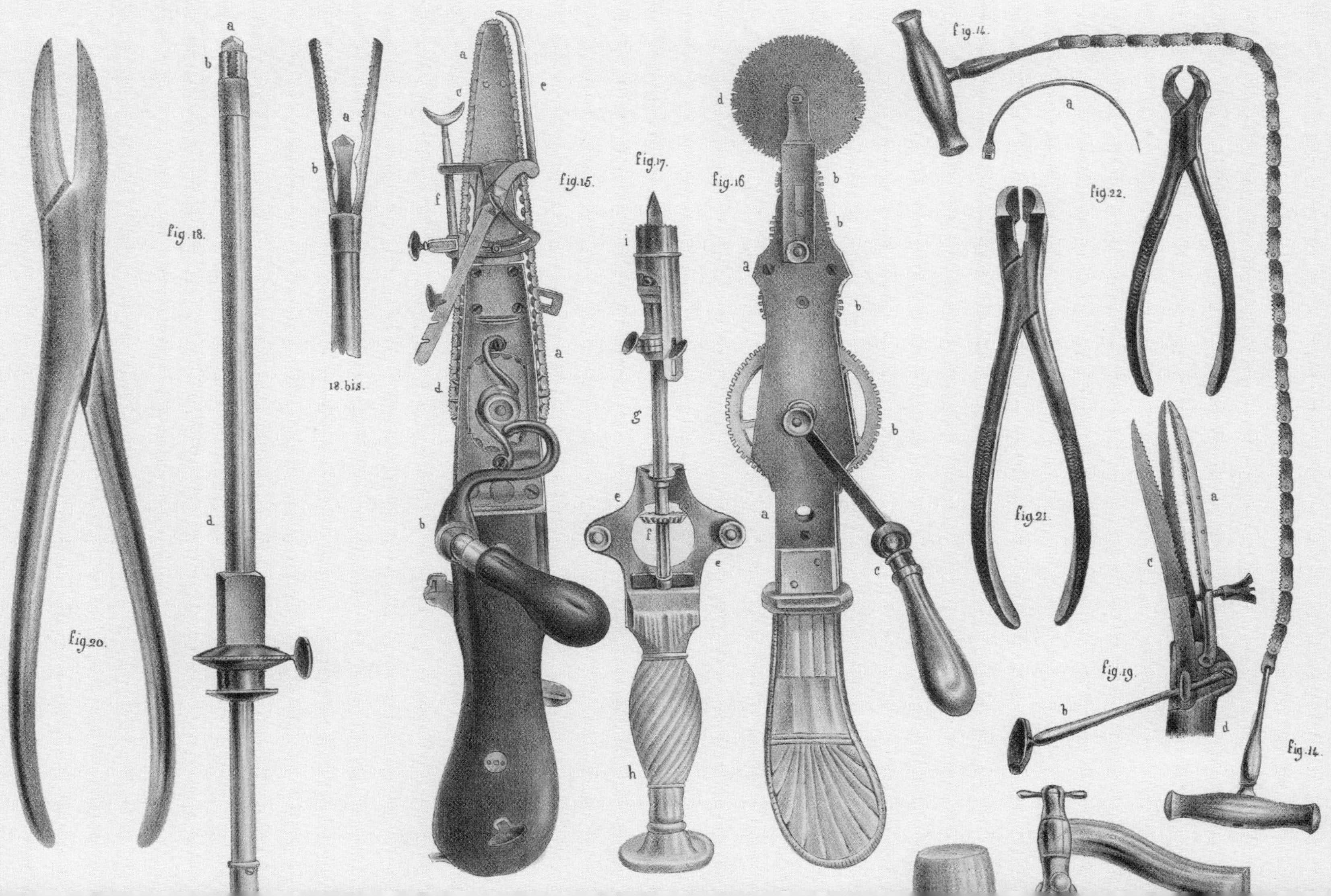

fig.20.

fig.18.

d

b

a

18.bis.

b

a

b

fig.15.

d

f

a

c

e

h

e

f

g

i

fig.17.

fig.16.

a

d

a

c

b

b

b

c

b

fig.14.

a

fig.21.

fig.22.

b

fig.19.

c

a

d

fig.14.

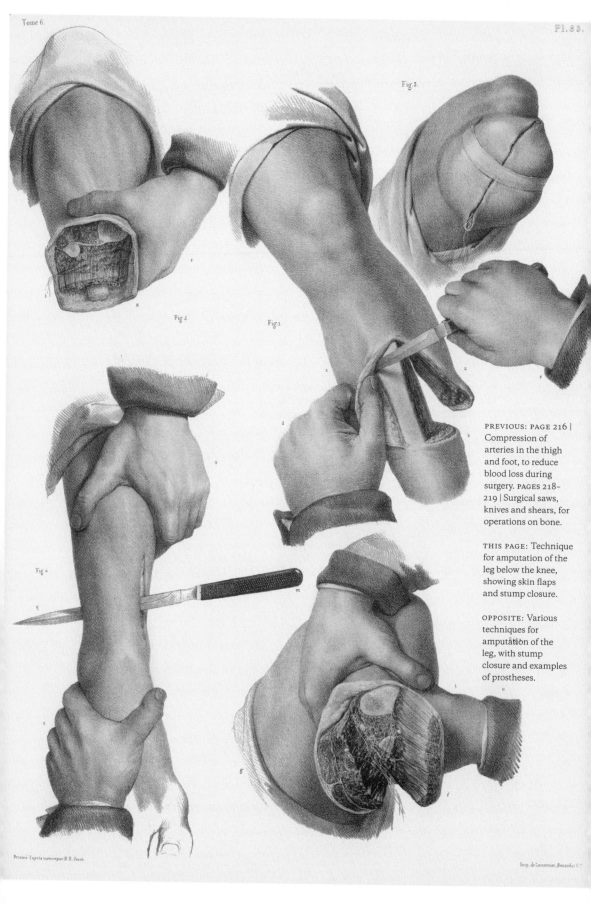

Fig. 3.

Fig. 5.

Fig. 1.

Fig. 4.

PREVIOUS: PAGE 216 |
Compression of
arteries in the thigh
and foot, to reduce
blood loss during
surgery. PAGES 218–
219 | Surgical saws,
knives and shears, for
operations on bone.

THIS PAGE: Technique
for amputation of the
leg below the knee,
showing skin flaps
and stump closure.

OPPOSITE: Various
techniques for
amputation of the
leg, with stump
closure and examples
of prostheses.

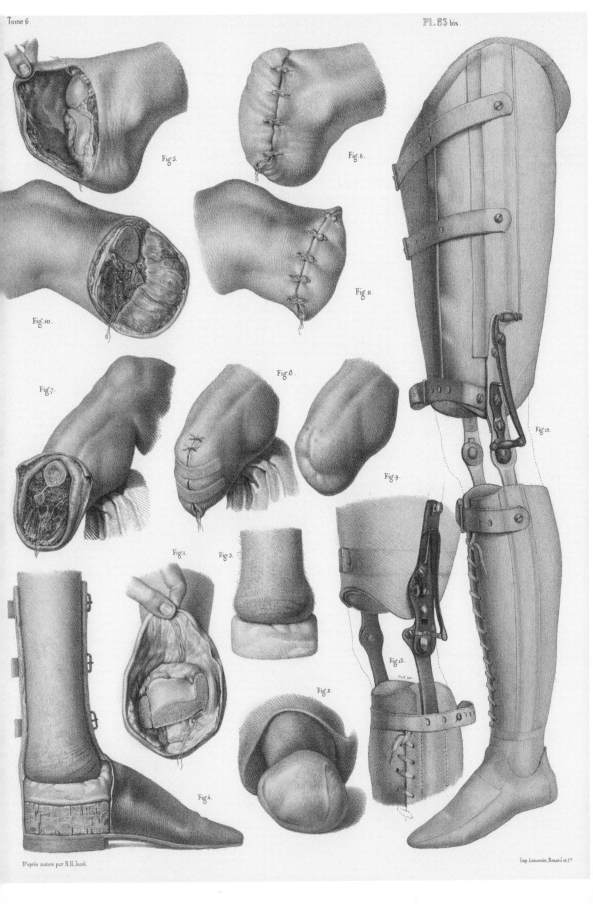

Pl. 85 bis.

Fig. 5.

Fig. 6.

Fig. 10.

Fig. 11.

Fig. 7.

Fig. 8.

Fig. 9.

Fig. 12.

Fig. 1.

Fig. 3.

Fig. 13.

Fig. 2.

Fig. 4.

D'après nature par N.H. Jacob.

Imp. Lemercier, Bénard et C.ie

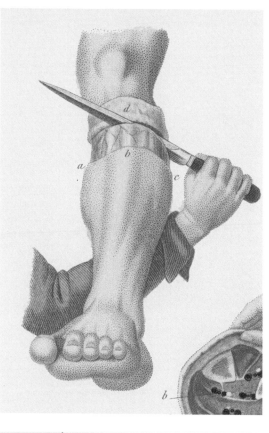

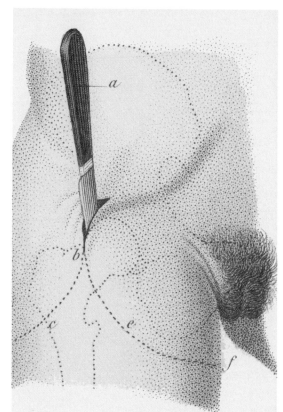

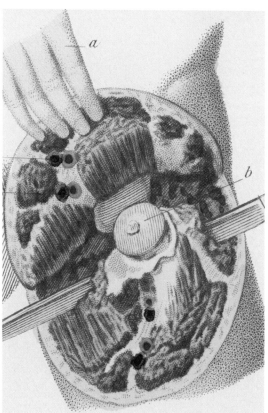

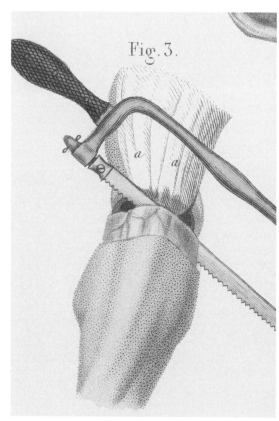

Fig. 3.

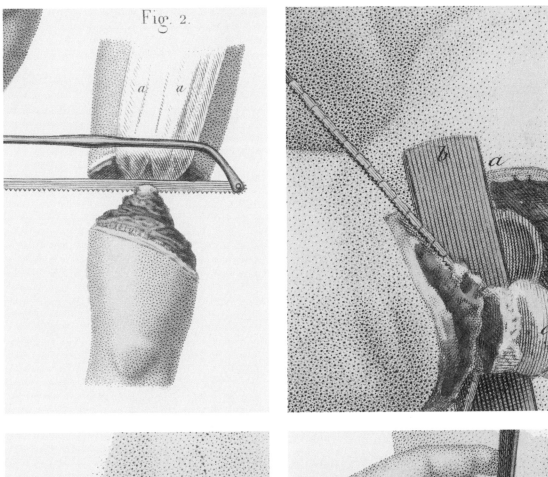

Fig. 2.

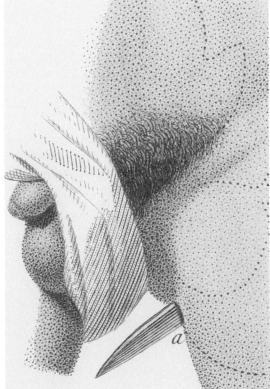

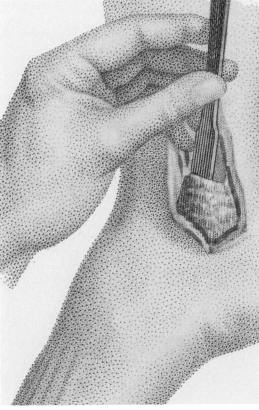

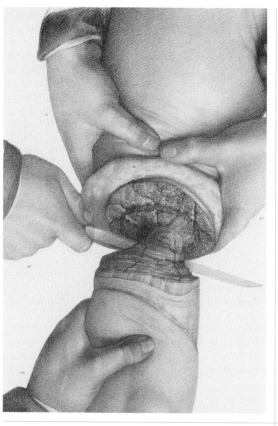

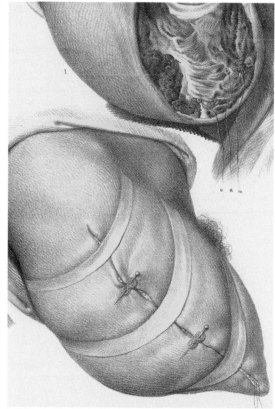

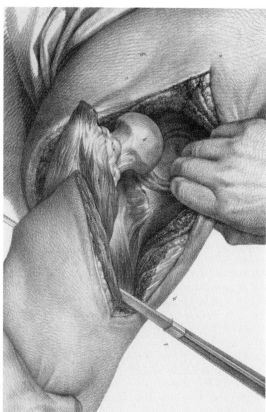

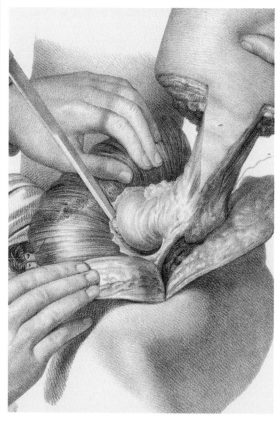

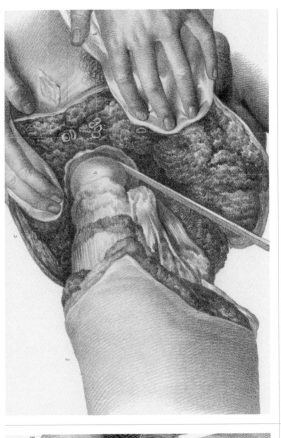

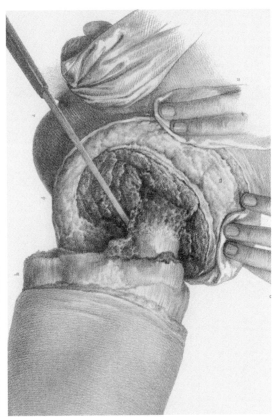

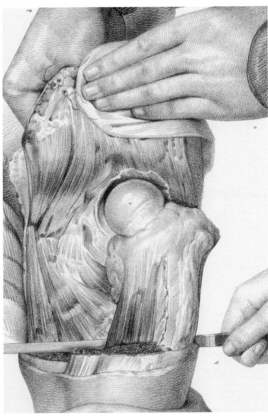

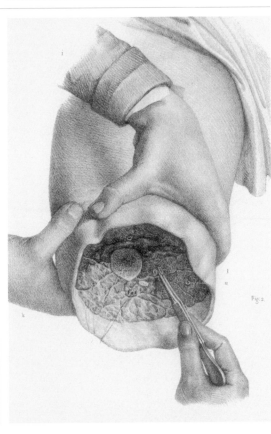

Fig. 2.

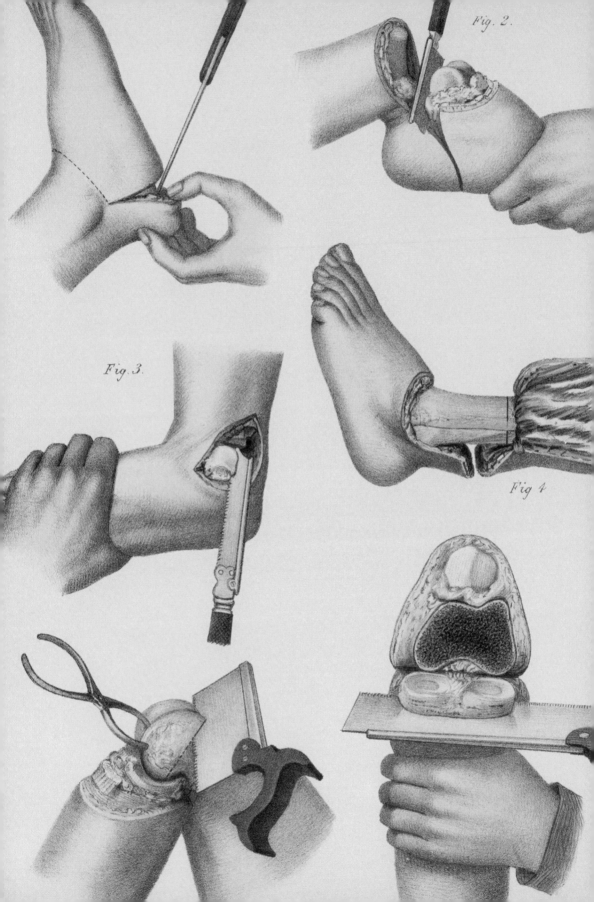

Fig. 2.

Fig. 3.

Fig 4

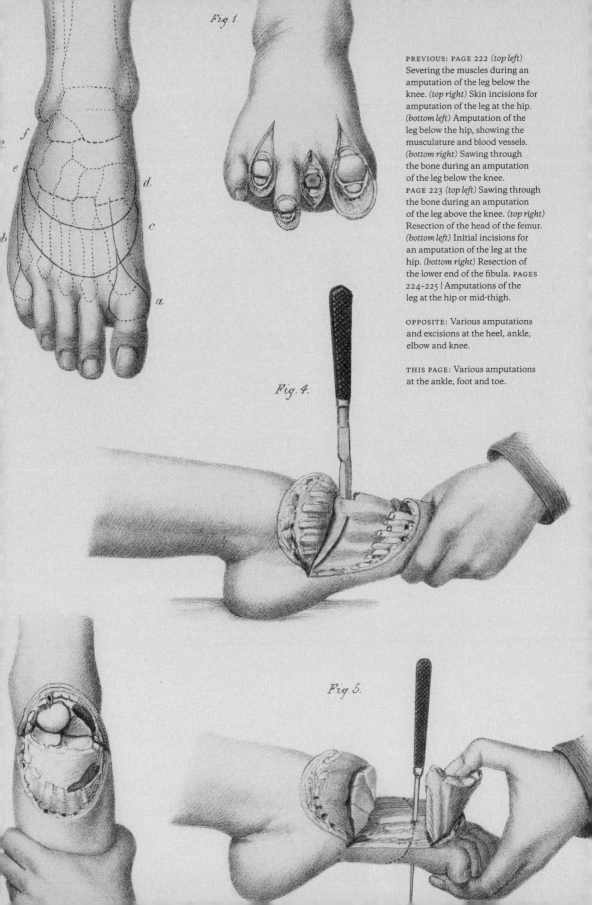

Fig. 1.

f
e
d
c
b
a

PREVIOUS: PAGE 222 (*top left*)
Severing the muscles during an
amputation of the leg below the
knee. (*top right*) Skin incisions for
amputation of the leg at the hip.
(*bottom left*) Amputation of the
leg below the hip, showing the
musculature and blood vessels.
(*bottom right*) Sawing through
the bone during an amputation
of the leg below the knee.
PAGE 223 (*top left*) Sawing through
the bone during an amputation
of the leg above the knee. (*top right*)
Resection of the head of the femur.
(*bottom left*) Initial incisions for
an amputation of the leg at the
hip. (*bottom right*) Resection of
the lower end of the fibula. PAGES
224–225 | Amputations of the
leg at the hip or mid-thigh.

OPPOSITE: Various amputations
and excisions at the heel, ankle,
elbow and knee.

THIS PAGE: Various amputations
at the ankle, foot and toe.

Fig. 4.

Fig. 5.

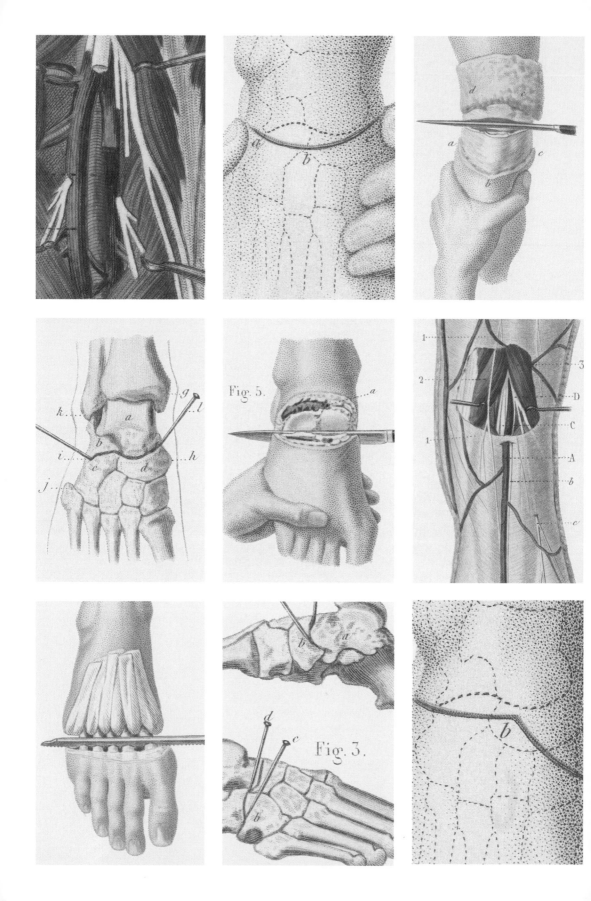

Fig. 5.

Fig. 3.

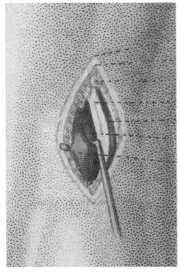

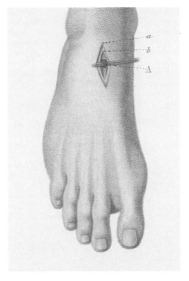

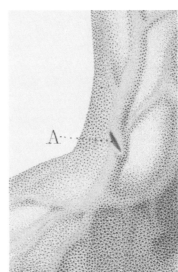

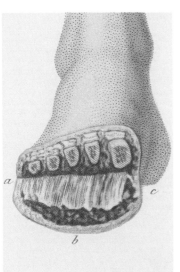

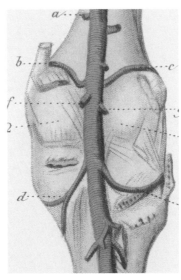

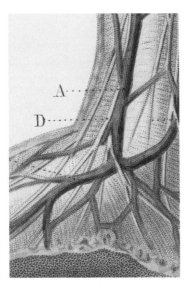

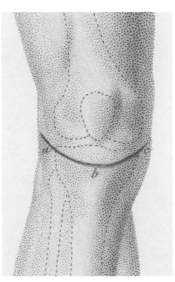

OPPOSITE: *(top left & centre right)* Surgical anatomy of the popliteal fossa, showing site for ligature of the popliteal artery. *(top centre)* Surface markers for amputation of the foot at the metatarsal bones. *(top right)* Amputation of the leg at the knee. *(centre left)* Skeletal anatomy for amputation of the foot at the metatarsal bones. *(centre)* Amputation of the foot at the metatarsal bones. *(bottom left)* Amputation of the foot at the metatarsophalangeal joints. *(bottom centre & right)* Skeletal anatomy for amputation of the foot.

THIS PAGE: *(top left)* Ligature of the popliteal artery. *(top centre)* Ligature of the radial and dorsalis pedis arteries. *(top right)* Incision of veins in the ankle. *(centre left)* Amputation of the toes. *(centre)* The branches of the popliteal artery. *(bottom left)* Veins in the ankle. *(bottom centre)* Surface markers for amputation of the leg at the tibiofemoral joint.

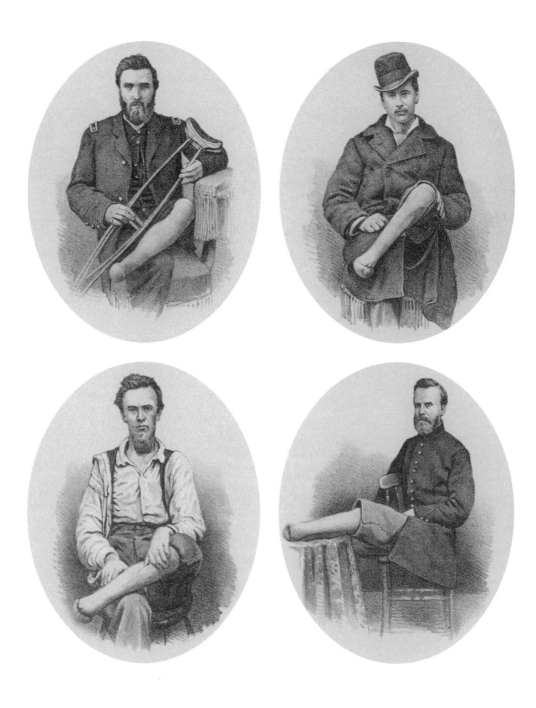

ABOVE: Four veterans of the American Civil War with amputations at the ankle joints. (*top left*) Lieutenant W. C. Weeks (*top right*) Private J. E. Ayers (*bottom left*) Private J. H. Short (*bottom right*) Private A. K. Russell.

OPPOSITE: A veteran of the American Civil War with his right leg amputated at the hip.

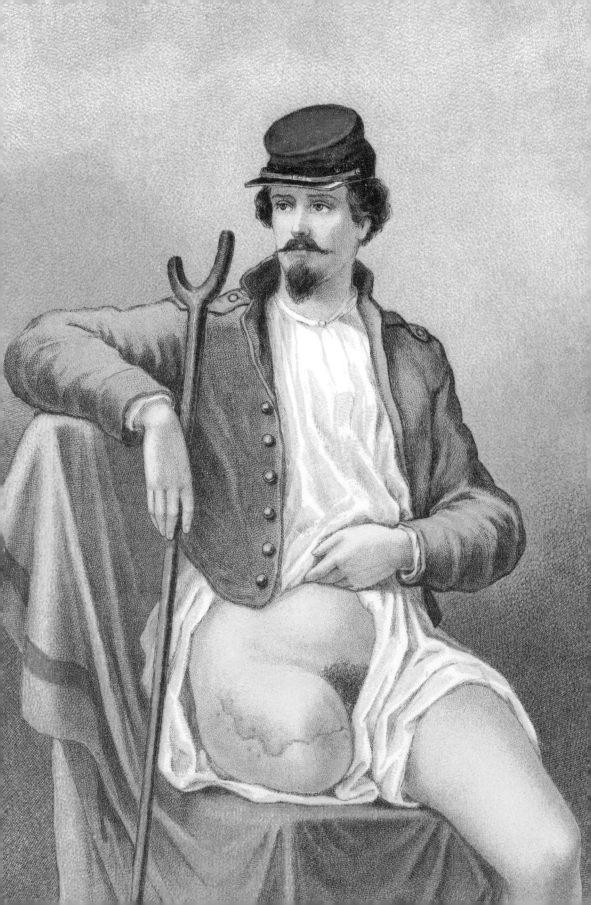

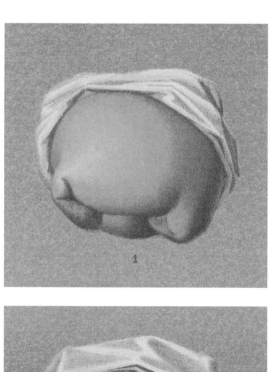

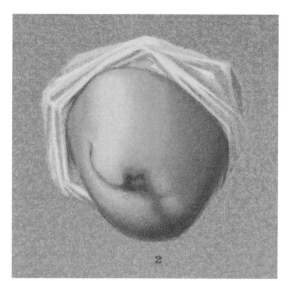

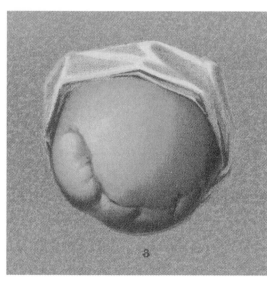

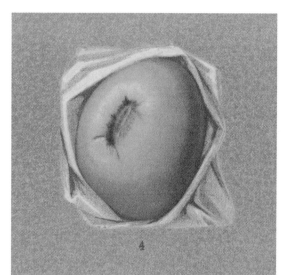

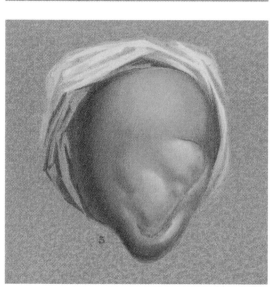

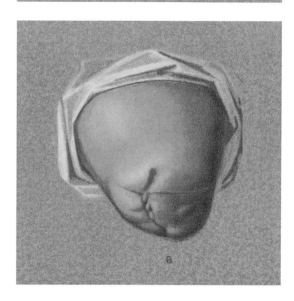

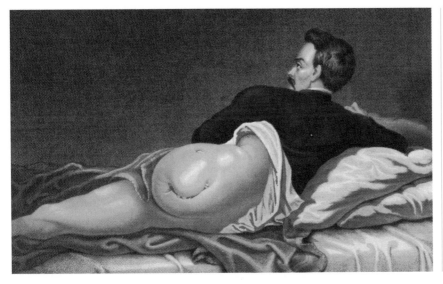

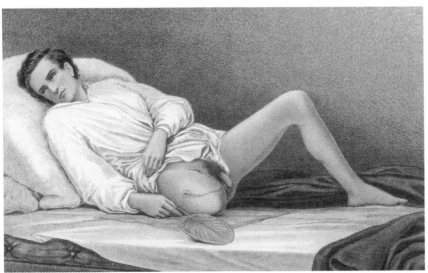

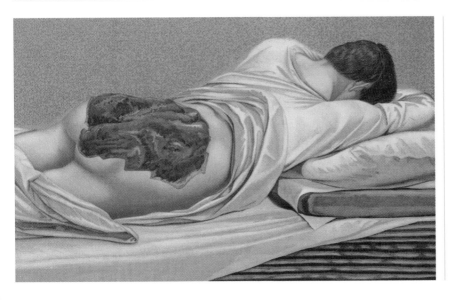

OPPOSITE: Healed thigh stumps after the amputation of the leg at mid-thigh by various techniques.

THIS PAGE: *(top & centre)* Amputation of the leg at the hip. *(bottom)* Laceration of the buttocks by a shell fragment.

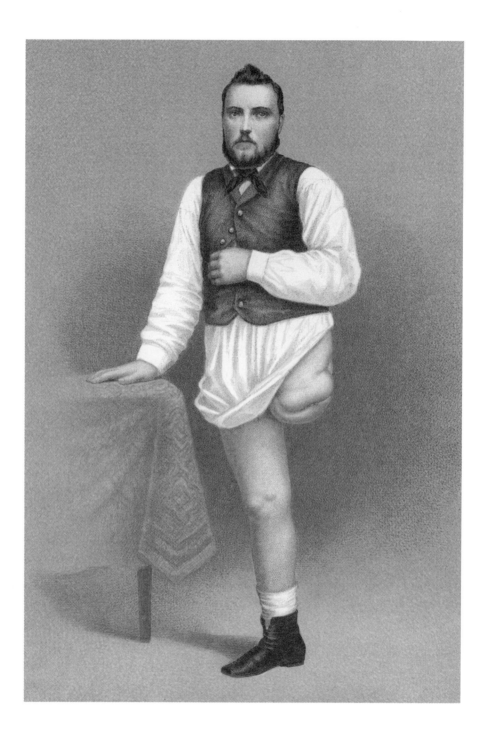

ABOVE & OPPOSITE: Re-amputation of the leg at the hip.

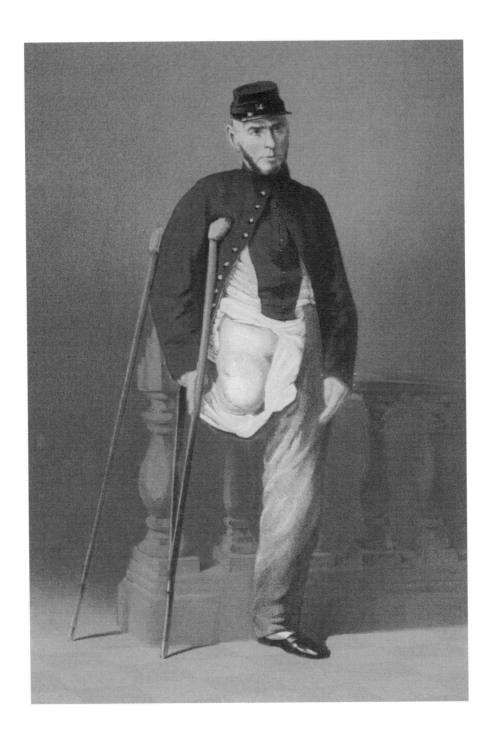

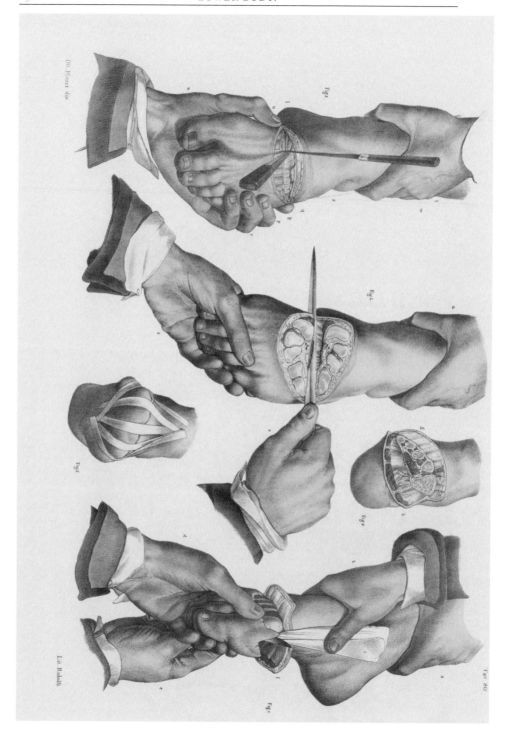

ABOVE: Amputation of the toes at the metatarsals.
OPPOSITE: Amputation of various toes, and amputation of the toes at the metatarsals.

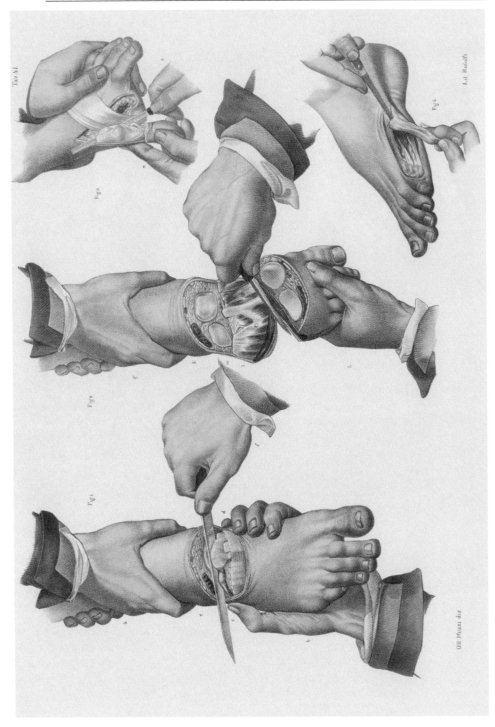

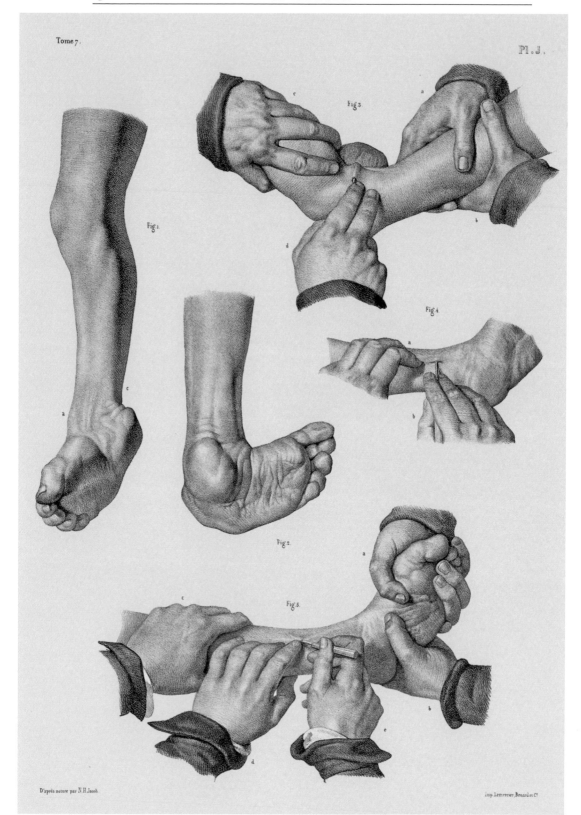

D'après nature par N. H. Jacob.

Imp. Lemercier, Benard et C.ⁱᵉ

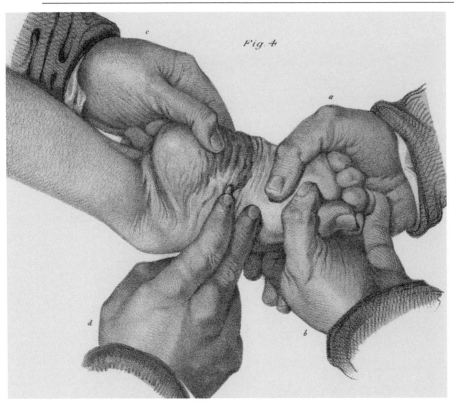

OPPOSITE:
Club foot, and a
corrective procedure.

THIS PAGE:
Subcutaneous
procedures to
correct club foot.

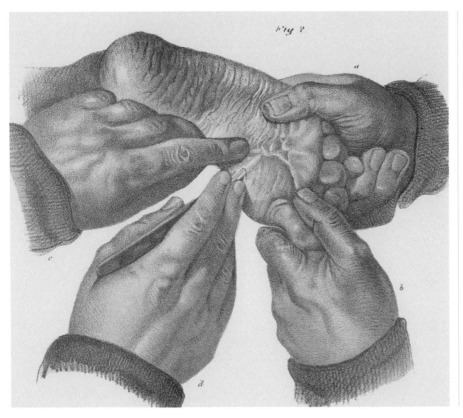

UNDER THE KNIFE: *The Patient's Perspective.*

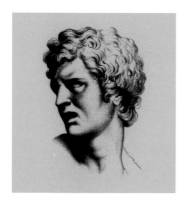

Fig. 1.

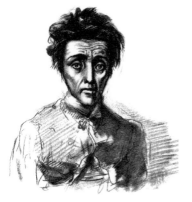

Fig. 2.

Having had surgery to sever scar tissue holding his right arm to his body—the consequence of a poorly healed injury he suffered in a Manchester cotton mill in the 1820s—eighteen-year-old Joseph Townend made the mistake of offering his uninjured left hand in greeting to his surgeon a day or two after the operation:

> *'Do you offer a gentleman your left hand?'*
> *Seizing my right hand, he dragged me off the*
> *bed into the middle of the room… With violence*
> *he struck at the same moment with one fist*
> *the knee, and with the other the elbow, sternly*
> *exclaiming 'Stand up, man; you have not your*
> *mother for your doctor now!' Immediately my*
> *leg and foot were covered with blood.*

Stories like this might be multiplied almost infinitely. Take, for instance, the work of the German surgeon Johann Friedrich Dieffenbach at the Charité Hospital in Berlin. On one hand, Dieffenbach spent his professional life finding surgical solutions to disfiguring contractures, squints and facial injuries. On the other, his drastic procedure for the treatment of stammering, developed in 1841 when the thought struck him 'that an incision carried completely through the root of the tongue might be useful in stuttering which had resisted other means of cure', resulted in a great deal of unnecessary suffering amongst his patients. Cutting a triangular wedge out of the root of the tongue—something he first tried on a thirteen-year-old boy who stuttered in German, French and Latin—produced, at best, ambiguous results, and inaugurated a fashion across Europe for similar procedures. His French and English colleagues hacked away at tongues, adenoids and even the skulls of their patients in what the *Lancet* deplored as 'a perfect mania for operating... [with] the frightful attendant haemorrhage, the great risk of losing the tongue, or life itself.'

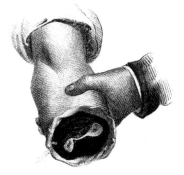

Fig. 3.

Histories of surgery from the patient's perspective are so often stories of suffering, its relief or—in these cases—its prolongation. Under the new surgical regimes established after Paris medicine, poor patients were not customers to be satisfied but sick bodies to be diagnosed and treated; their voices were no longer a source of clinical information and interpretation. In this sense patients became, for the most part, silent partners in nineteenth-century surgery.

Joanna Bourke has argued that with hospital-based practice and disease-orientated diagnosis came a 'thinning' of the language around pain, reflecting the marginalization of patients' experiences.[1] As we saw in *The Smart of the Knife: Surgery & War* (E; pages 160–165) Victorian practitioners and patients were using new and vivid ways to describe pain, many of them drawn from the language of war, but it is certainly true that hospital case notes tended to record only the severity and not the texture of pain. Even after the introduction of anaesthesia, patients might find themselves suffering in silence, as in the case of Mary Roesly, who underwent several amputations in the 1860s:

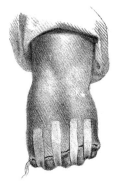

Fig. 4.

[1] Joanna Bourke, *The Story of Pain: From Prayer to Painkillers*, Oxford University Press, 2014.

> *I stood this operation with some fortitude, as it elicited the remark from several physicians that I was 'courageous', yet the reader will understand that such remarks are generally made to render the sometime timid brave, but my silent sufferings were terrible to me.*

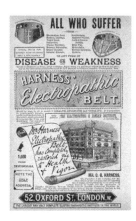

Fig. 5.

Depending on who was suffering and in what context, the meaning of silent suffering could be strikingly different: it might be a courageous attempt to spare the feelings of loved ones, a trial of faith or manhood, or even a kind of antisocial cowardice. From the perspective of surgeons, too, the meaning of pain itself changed across the nineteenth century, particularly after the advent of anaesthesia. Christopher Lawrence has observed that, for surgeons at the end of the century:

> If [pain] had a purpose it was to teach people, especially poor people, to be grateful to medicine, not God .[2]

This was not just a matter of surgeons exercising their newfound authority over patients. As surgery became a treatment that patients might choose, rather than a last resort, so some surgeons began to devise operations to cure diseases that (in Ann Dally's words) 'existed only in the minds of the doctors and their patients'.[3] The Harley Street surgeon Sir William Arbuthnot Lane became notorious for charging patients large sums to correct 'dropped organs', and others offered surgical cures for 'autointoxication', 'chronic intestinal stasis' or 'focal sepsis'. One reading of this is as nothing more than avaricious quackery, as in the caption to an 1877 *Punch* cartoon:

FIRST SURGEON: *What did you operate on Jones for?*
SECOND SURGEON: *A hundred pounds.*
FIRST SURGEON: *No, I mean what had he got?*
SECOND SURGEON: *A hundred pounds.*

This keenness also reflects the growing desire of surgeons to turn all of medicine into a surgical jurisdiction, and make surgery a cure for all diseases. What Elizabeth Blackwell (one of the first women to qualify as a physician) described as the 'itch to cut' was also manifest in attempts to control women's behaviour through surgery. From 1872, the American surgeon Robert Battey performed what

[2] Christopher Lawrence, 1992.

[3] Ann Dally, *Fantasy Surgery, 1880–1930*, Rodopi, 1996.

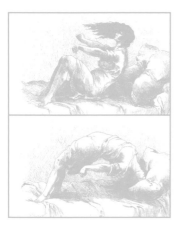

Fig. 6.

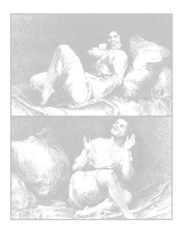

Fig. 7.

he called 'normal ovariotomies', removing healthy ovaries in the hope of relieving female symptoms of 'hystero-epilepsy' or 'ovariomania'. His London contemporary Isaac Baker Brown performed dozens of clitoridectomies without consent on women whose husbands had complained they were oversexed or had been masturbating.

Even before the emergence of anaesthesia, women had become the subjects of experimental surgery. From 1809, the Kentucky surgeon Ephraim McDowell was successfully removing massive ovarian tumours, and in Alabama James Marion Sims developed a procedure to repair fistulas between the bladder and the vagina. Stories about the women who underwent these surgeries provide flashes of insight into their experiences. Jane Todd Crawford, McDowell's first surviving patient, sang hymns to blur the pain during her twenty-five-minute ordeal, and most of Sims' early patients were slave women who had developed fistulas after long, untended labours or a dozen or more pregnancies. Surgery for women at the end of the nineteenth century might have been less painful, but it could still be appallingly disfiguring. The radical mastectomy developed by William Halsted at Johns Hopkins Hospital in the 1890s removed not only the entire breast but also the lymph nodes, chest muscles and even parts of the ribcage.

With this in mind, it seems appropriate to end our story where many histories of surgery begin, with one of the most famous descriptions of surgery in the age before anaesthesia. In 1811, the novelist Fanny Burney underwent a mastectomy for breast cancer with the French military surgeon Dominique-Jean Larrey, and later wrote a long letter to her sister in which she described the surgery. The passages recounting the operation itself are well known:

> Yet—when the dreadful steel was plunged into the breast—cutting through veins—arteries—flesh— nerves — I needed no injunctions not to restrain

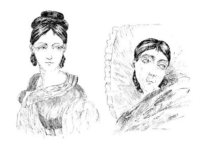

Fig. 8.

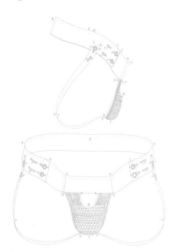

Fig. 9.

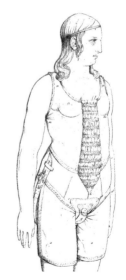

Fig. 10.

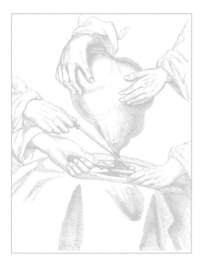

Fig. 11.

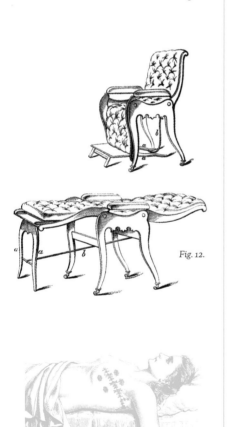

Fig. 12.

Fig. 13.

my cries. I began a scream that lasted unintermittingly during the whole time of the incision—& I almost marvel that it rings not in my Ears still? so excruciating was the agony. When the wound was made, & the instrument was withdrawn, the pain seemed undiminished, for the air that suddenly rushed into those delicate parts felt like a mass of minute but sharp & forked poniards, that were tearing the edges of the wound. I concluded the operation was over—Oh no! presently the terrible cutting was renewed—& worse than ever, to separate the bottom, the foundation of this dreadful gland from the parts to which it adhered—Again all description would be baffled—yet again all was not over,—Dr. Larry rested but his own hand, &—Oh heaven!—I then felt the knife (rack)ling against the breast bone—scraping it!

Less familiar is Burney's deeply moving account of her condition almost a year later:

Not for days, not for Weeks, but for Months I could not speak of this terrible business without nearly again going through it! I could not think of it with impunity! I was sick, I was disordered by a single question— even now, 9 months after it is over, I have a headache from going on with the account! and this miserable account, which I began 3 Months ago, at least, I dare not revise, nor read, the recollection is still so painful.

Surgical histories that revolve around great surgeons and their pioneering operations do so at the risk of excluding other stories—most importantly, those of patients and the long aftermath of surgery. The memory of pain and its persistence, the task of learning to live in an altered, perhaps diminished body, and this feeling of a compromise between survival and wholeness are what surgery has meant for so many across the centuries.

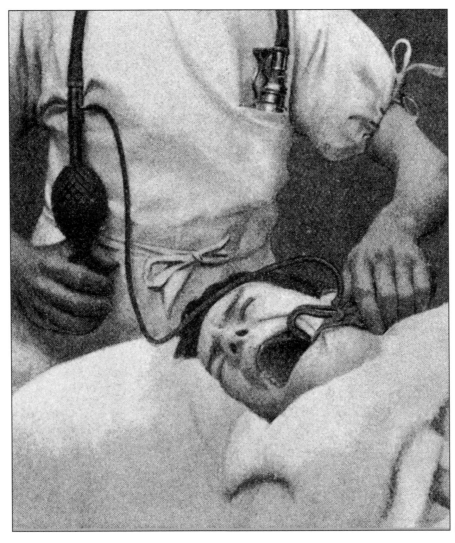

Fig. 14.

FIG. 1: *From Classical times Western artists took a close interest in capturing states of extreme emotion: here the French artist Charles Le Brun (1619-1690) depicts acute pain.* FIG. 2: *This 1892 lithograph of a female asylum patient suffering from melancholia seems to capture the exhausting consequences of pain.* FIGS. 3&4: *Even after the introduction of anaesthesia, amputations such as this could leave patients suffering severe chronic pain.* FIG. 5: *These 'therapeutic belts', sold by the Electropathic and Zander Institute in the 1880s and 1890s, were claimed to relieve all kinds of chronic pain along with menstrual disorders, impotence and obesity.* FIGS. 6&7: *Two stages—'clownism' and 'passionate attitudes'—in the complex classification of female 'grand hysterie' developed by the French neurologist Jean-Martin Charcot (1825-1893).* FIG. 8: *Changing sexual attitudes in the nineteenth century led physicians to censure masturbation as a waste of vital energy. This French engraving from 1836 shows the purported effects of masturbation on a fifteen-year-old girl.* FIGS. 9&10: *Two early nineteenth-century French designs for corsets intended to stop their wearers masturbating.* FIG. 11: *Removal of a large ovarian cyst, from an 1872 surgical treatise.* FIG. 12: *This chair for obstetrical surgery was designed by the American surgeon James Marion Sims (1813-1883).* FIG. 13: *Early mastectomies for breast cancer frequently involved the removal not only of the breast but also of much of the surrounding tissue.* FIG. 14: *At the beginning of the twentieth century surgeons used gags such as this to hold the mouth open during facial or oral surgery.*

FURTHER READING

WEBSITES:

Brought to Life: Exploring the History of Medicine—www. sciencemuseum.org.uk/ broughttolife.aspx
—
Dream Anatomy— www.nlm.nih.gov/ dreamanatomy
—
London's Museums of Health and Medicine— www.medicalmuseums.org
—
Medical History: An International Journal for the History of Medicine and Related Sciences—journals. cambridge.org/action/ displayJournal?jid=MDH
—
Morbid Anatomy— morbidanatomy.blogspot. com
—
National Library of Medicine— www.nlm.nih.gov
—
Royal College of Surgeons of England— www.rcseng.ac.uk
—
Wellcome Images— wellcomeimages.org
—
Wellcome Library— wellcomelibrary.org
—
Wellcome Trust— www.wellcome.ac.uk

OVERVIEWS:

William F. Bynum *et al, The Western Medical Tradition: 1800 to 2000,* Cambridge University Press, 2006.
—
Harry M. Collins, 'Dissecting surgery: forms of life depersonalised', *Social Studies of Science* 24, 1994, 311-333.
—
Lawrence Conrad *et al, The Western Medical Tradition: 800 BC to AD 1800,* Cambridge University Press, 1995. [Hard copy]
—
Roger French, 'The anatomical tradition', in William F. Bynum & Roy Porter (eds), *Companion Encyclopaedia of the History of Medicine,* Routledge, 1993, vol 1, 81-101.
—
Christopher Lawrence (ed), *Medical Theory, Surgical Practice: Studies in the History of Surgery,* Routledge, 1992.
—
Christopher Lawrence, 'Medical minds, surgical bodies', in Christopher Lawrence & Steven Shapin (eds), *Science Incarnate: Historical Embodiments of Natural Knowledge,* University of Chicago Press, 156-201.
—
Roy Porter, *The Greatest Benefit to Mankind: A Medical History of Humanity from Antiquity to the Present,* Harper Collins, 1997.

MEDIEVAL & EARLY MODERN SURGERY:

A. L. Beier, 'Seventeenth-century English surgery: the casebook of Joseph Binns', in Christopher Lawrence (ed), *Medical Theory, Surgical Practice: Studies in the History of Surgery,* Routledge, 1992.
—
Robert Jutte, 'A seventeenth-century German barber-surgeon and his patients', *Medical History* 33, 1989, 184-198.
—
Ghislaine Lawrence, 'Surgery (traditional)', in William F Bynum & Roy Porter (eds), *Companion Encyclopaedia of the History of Medicine,* Routledge, 1993, vol 2, 961-983.
—
Vivian Nutton, 'Humanist surgery', in Andrew Wear *et al* (eds), *The Medical Renaissance of the Sixteenth Century,* Cambridge University Press, 1985, 75-99.
—
Vivian Nutton, 'Medicine in medieval western Europe, 1000-1500', in Lawrence Conrad *et al, The Western Medical Tradition: 800 BC to AD 1800,* Cambridge University Press, 1995, section on 'Apothecaries and surgeons', 159-163.
—
Margaret Pelling, 'Appearance and reality: barber-surgeons, the body and disease', in A. L. Beier & Roger Findlay (eds),

London 1500-1700: The Making of the Metropolis, Longman, 1985, 82-112.

—

Andrew Wear, 'Medicine in early modern Europe, 1500-1700', in Lawrence Conrad et al, The Western Medical Tradition: 800 BC to AD 1800, Cambridge University Press, 1995, section on 'Surgery', 292-297.

EIGHTEENTH-CENTURY SURGERY:

William F. Bynum & Roy Porter (eds), William Hunter and the Eighteenth-century Medical World, Cambridge University Press, 2002.

—

Toby Gelfand, Professionalising Modern Medicine: Paris Surgeons and Medical Science and Institutions in the Eighteenth Century, Greenwood Press, 1982.

—

Wendy Moore, The Knife Man: Blood, Body-snatching and the Birth of Modern Surgery, Bantam, 2006.

—

Roy Porter, 'The eighteenth century', in Lawrence Conrad et al, The Western Medical Tradition: 800 BC to AD 1800, Cambridge University Press, 1995, section on 'Surgery', 434-449.

—

Owsei Temkin, 'The role of surgery in the rise of modern medical thought', Bulletin of the History of

Medicine 25, 1951, 248-259. (Reprinted in The Double Face of Janus and Other Essays in the History of Medicine, Johns Hopkins University Press, 1977, 487-496)

—

Philip K. Wilson, 'Acquiring surgical know-how: occupational and lay instruction in early eighteenth-century England', in Roy Porter (ed), The Popularisation of Medicine, Routledge, 1992, 42-71.

NINETEENTH-CENTURY SURGERY:

William F. Bynum, Science and the Practice of Medicine in the Nineteenth Century, Cambridge University Press, 1994.

—

Michel Foucault, The Birth of the Clinic: An Archaeology of Medical Perception [1963], trans. Alan Sheridan, Tavistock, 1973.

—

Thomas Schlich, 'The emergence of modern surgery', in Deborah Brunton (ed), Medicine Transformed: Health, Disease and Society in Europe, 1800-1939, Manchester, 2004, 61-91.

—

Peter Stanley, For Fear of Pain: British Surgery 1790-1850, Rodopi, 2003.

—

Ulrich Tröhler, 'Surgery (modern)', in William F. Bynum & Roy Porter (eds),

Companion Encyclopaedia of the History of Medicine, Routledge, 1993, vol 2, 984-1028.

ANAESTHESIA:

Joanna Bourke, The Story of Pain: From Prayer to Painkillers, Oxford University Press, 2014.

—

Margaret C. Jacob & Michael J. Sauter, 'Why did Humphry Davy and associates not pursue the pain-alleviating effects of nitrous oxide?', Journal of the History of Medicine and Allied Sciences 57, 2002, 161-176.

—

Martin S. Pernick, A Calculus of Suffering: Pain, Professionalism and Anaesthesia in Nineteenth-century America, Columbia University Press, 1985.

—

Stephanie J. Snow, Operations Without Pain: The Practice and Science of Anaesthesia in Victorian Britain, Palgrave Macmillan, 2006.

—

Stephanie J. Snow, Blessed Days of Anaesthesia: How Anaesthetics Changed the World, Oxford University Press, 2008.

—

Alison Winter, Mesmerised: Powers of Mind in Victorian Britain, University of Chicago Press, 1998.

ANTISEPSIS
& THE HOSPITAL:

M. Anne Crowther &
Marguerite W. Dupree,
*Medical Lives in the Age
of Surgical Revolution*,
Cambridge University
Press, 2007.
—
N. J. Fox, 'Scientific
theory choice and social
structure: the case of
Joseph Lister's antisepsis,
humoral theory and
asepsis', *History of Science*
26, 1988, 367-397.
—
Lindsay Granshaw,
'The hospital', in William
F. Bynum & Roy Porter
(eds), *Companion
Encyclopaedia of the History
of Medicine*, Routledge,
1993, vol 2, 1180-1203.
—
Lindsay Granshaw, '"Upon
this principle I have based a
practice": the development
and reception of antisepsis
in Britain, 1867-90', in
John V. Pickstone (ed),
*Medical Innovations in
Historical Perspective*,
Macmillan, 1992, 17-46.
—
Anna Greenwood, 'Lawson
Tait and opposition to germ
theory: defining science in
surgical practice', *Journal
of the History of Medicine
and Allied Sciences*, 53,
1998, 99-131.
—
David Hamilton, 'The
nineteenth-century surgical
revolution—antisepsis or
better nutrition?', *Bulletin
of the History of Medicine* 56,
1982, 30-40.

Christopher Lawrence &
Richard Dixey, 'Practising
on principle: Joseph Lister
and the germ theories of
disease', in Christopher
Lawrence (ed), *Medical
Theory, Surgical Practice:
Studies in the History of
Surgery*, Routledge,
1992, 153-215.
—
T. H. Pennington,
'Listerism, its decline
and its persistence: the
introduction of aseptic
surgical techniques in
three British teaching
hospitals, 1890-99',
Medical History 39,
1995, 35-60.
—
Charles Rosenberg,
'Florence Nightingale on
contagion: the hospital
as moral universe', in
*Explaining Epidemics and
Other Studies in the History
of Medicine*, Cambridge
University Press, 1992,
90-108.
—
Christine Stevenson,
'Medicine and architecture',
in William F. Bynum & Roy
Porter (eds), *Companion
Encyclopaedia of the History
of Medicine*, Routledge,
1993, vol 2, 1495-1519.

ASEPSIS & THE
OPERATING THEATRE:

Ken Arnold & Thomas
Söderqvist, 'Medical
instruments in museums:
immediate impressions
and historical meanings',
Isis 102, 2011, 718-729.
Ghislaine Lawrence,

'The ambiguous artefact:
surgical instruments
and the surgical past',
in Christopher Lawrence
(ed), *Medical Theory,
Surgical Practice: Studies
in the History of Surgery*,
Routledge, 1992, 295-314.
—
Thomas Schlich, 'Surgery,
science and modernity:
operating rooms and
laboratories as spaces
of control', *History of
Science* 45, 2007, 231-256.
—
Thomas Schlich, 'Asepsis
and bacteriology: a
realignment of surgery
and laboratory science',
Medical History 56, 2012,
308-334.
—
Carsten Timmerman
& Julie Anderson (eds),
*Devices and Designs:
Medical Technologies
in Historical Perspective*,
Palgrave Macmillan, 2006.

SURGERY & NURSING:

Mark Bostridge, *Florence
Nightingale: The Woman
and Her Legend*, Viking
Books, 2008.
—
Ludmila Jordanova, *Sexual
Visions: Images of Gender in
Science and Medicine Between
the Eighteenth and Twentieth
Centuries*, University of
Wisconsin Press, 1989.
—
Christopher Maggs, 'A
general history of nursing:
1800-1900', in William F.
Bynum & Roy Porter (eds),
Companion Encyclopaedia

of the History of Medicine, Routledge, 1993, vol 2, 1309-1328.

—

Charles Rosenberg, 'Florence Nightingale on contagion: the hospital as moral universe', in *Explaining Epidemics and Other Studies in the History of Medicine*, Cambridge University Press, 1992, 90-108.

SURGERY & WAR:

Roger Cooter, 'War and modern medicine', in William F. Bynum & Roy Porter (eds), *Companion Encyclopaedia of the History of Medicine*, Routledge, 1993, 1536-1563.

—

Roger Cooter, *Surgery and Society in Peace and War: Orthopaedics and the Organisation of Modern Medicine 1880-1948*, Macmillan, 1993.

—

Roger Cooter, Mark Harrison, & Steve Sturdy (eds), *War, Medicine and Modernity*, Sutton, 1998.

Mark Harrison, 'Medicine and the management of modern warfare', *History of Science* 34, 1996, 379-410.

—

Matthew H. Kaufman, *Surgeons at War: Medical Arrangements for the Treatment of the Sick and Wounded in the British Army During the Late 18th and 19th Centuries*, Greenwood, 2001.

Matthew H. Kaufman,

The Regius Chair of Military Surgery in the University of Edinburgh, 1806-55, Rodopi, 2003.

TEACHING & ORGANIZING SURGERY:

L. S. Jacyna, 'The laboratory and the clinic: the impact of pathology on surgical diagnosis in the Glasgow Western Infirmary, 1875-1920', *Bulletin of the History of Medicine* 62, 1988, 384-406.

—

Christopher Lawrence, 'Incommunicable knowledge: science, technology and the clinical art in Britain, 1850-1914', *Journal of Contemporary History* 20, 1985, 503-520.

—

Ruth Richardson, *Death, Dissection and the Destitute*, Routledge, 1987.

—

George Weisz, *Divide and Conquer: A Comparative History of Medical Specialisation*, Oxford University Press, 2005.

THE STATUS OF SURGERY:

Sally Frampton, 'Applause and Amazement': Social Identity and the London Surgical Elite, 1880-1905, University of London MA thesis, 2008.

—

L. S. Jacyna, 'Images of John Hunter in the

nineteenth century', *History of Science*, 1983, 85-108.

—

Christopher Lawrence, 'Democratic, divine and heroic: the history and historiography of surgery', in *Medical Theory, Surgical Practice: Studies in the History of Surgery*, Routledge, 1992, 1-47.

—

Thomas Schlich, 'How gods and saints became transplant surgeons: the scientific article as a model for the writing of history', *History of Science* 33, 1995, 311-331.

PATIENTS' EXPERIENCES OF SURGERY:

Joanna Bourke, *The Story of Pain: From Prayer to Painkillers*, Oxford University Press, 2014.

—

Ann Dally, *Fantasy Surgery, 1880-1930*, Rodopi, 1996.

—

Ann Dally, *Women Under the Knife: A History of Surgery*, Routledge, 1991.

—

Roy Porter, 'Pain and suffering', in William F. Bynum & Roy Porter (eds), *Companion Encyclopaedia of the History of Medicine*, Routledge, 1993, vol 2, 1574-1591.

—

Stephanie J. Snow, *Blessed Days of Anaesthesia: How Anaesthetics Changed the World*, Oxford University Press, 2008.

PICTURE

CREDITS

ALL IMAGES COURTESY OF WELLCOME LIBRARY,
LONDON, UNLESS STATED OTHERWISE.
t = top, **r** = right, **b** = bottom, **l** = left, **c** = centre

1 [Small bow-frame amputation saw, from Hamonic collection] *c.* 1580, photograph; **2** Claude Bernard & Charles Huette, *Précis iconographique de médecine opératoire et d'anatomie chirurgicale*, Paris, 1848, pl. 2; **4-5** Jean Baptiste Marc Bourgery & Nicolas Henri Jacob, *Iconografia d'anatomia chirurgica e di medicina operatoria*, Florence, 1841, vol. 1, pl. 14; **6** Bourgery & Jacob, *Iconografia d'anatomia*, 1841, vol. 1, pl. 14; **7** Bourgery & Jacob, *Iconografia d'anatomia*, 1841, vol. 1, pl. 15; **8-9** Bourgery & Jacob, *Iconografia d'anatomia*, 1841, vol. 2, pl. N; **11** Joseph Maclise , *Surgical Anatomy*, London, 1856, pl. xxi; **13** Bernard & Huette, 1848, pl. 26; **14** Johann Vesling, *Syntagma anatomicum*, Padua, 1647, frontispiece; **17** Johannes de Ketham, *Fasciculus Medicinae*, Venice, 1493; **20** Claudius (Pseudo) Galen, *Anathomia*, mid-15th century, folio 53 verso; **21** Aurelius Cornelius Celsus, *De Medicina libri octo*, 1746, frontispiece, reproduced in R. Burgess, *Portraits of doctors & scientists in the Wellcome Institute*, London, 1973; **22** Unknown after Husayn Bihzad, [Rhazes, a physician, examines a kneeling boy], colour process print; **24 l** Georg Bartisch, *Opthalmodouleia. Das ist Augendienst*, Dresden, 1535, folio 218 recto; **24 r** Bartisch, 1535, folio 186 verso; **25 l** Bartisch, 1535, folio 181 vers o; **25 r** Bartisch, 1535, folio 201 verso; **26** *Arzneibuch*, *c.* 1675, pp. 83-84; **27** *Arzneibuch*, *c.* 1675, pp. 69-70; **28** Mondino dei Luzzi & Guido da Vigevano, *Anatomies...*, Pavia, 1478, reproduced in Ernest Wickersheimer, *Anatomies de Mondino de Luzzi et de Guido de Vigevano*, Paris, 1926, fig. vi; **29 l** [English folding almanac in Latin], *c.* 1415-1420; **29 r** Unknown, [Zodiac Man], Iran, *c.* 12th-14th century, watercolour painting; **30** *Apocalypsis S. Johannis cum glossis et Vita S. Johannis; Ars Moriendi, etc.*, *c.* 1420, folio 41 recto; **31 l** [Armenian manuscript], 1795, frontispiece; **31 r** Heymando de Veteri Busco, *Ars Computistica*, 1488, folio 22 recto; **32** Andreas Vesalius, *De Humani Corporis Fabrica*, 1543, book II, p. 174; **33** William Clowes, *A Profitable and Necessarie Book of Observations, for All Those that are Burned with the Flame of Gun-Powder, etc...*, London, 1637; **34** Thomas Johnson, *The workes of that famous chirurgion Ambrose Parey translated out of Latine and compared with the French*, London, 1634, frontispiece; **35 all** Ambroise Paré, *La methode curative des playes, et fractures de la teste humaine. Avec les pourtraits des instruments necessaires pour la curation d'icelles*, Paris, 1561; **36 all** Ambroise Paré, *Instrumenta chyrurgiae et icones anathomicae*, Paris, 1564; **37 all** Paré, 1564; **39** J. June, [The march of the medical militants to the siege of Warwick-Lane-Castle], 1768, coloured etching; **40** artist unknown, [William Cheselden giving an anatomical demonstration to six spectators in the anatomy-theatre of the Barber-Surgeons' Company, London], *c.* 1730-1740, oil painting; **45** Ernest Board, [The surgeon Robert Liston demonstrating the amputation of a male patient's leg], *c.* 1912, painting; **46** Jean Baptiste Marc Bourgery & Nicolas Henri Jacob, *Traité complet de l'anatomie de l'homme comprenant la médecine opératoire ...avec planches lithographiées ...*, Paris, 1839, vol. 6, pl. 18; **48-49** Bourgery & Jacob, *Iconografia d'anatomia*, 1841, vol. 2, pl. 22 bis.; **50** Bourgery & Jacob, *Traité complet de l'anatomie de l'homme*, 1844, vol. 3, pl. 16; **51** Bourgery & Jacob, *Traité complet de l'anatomie de l'homme*, 1844, vol. 3, pl. 35; **52 t** Bourgery & Jacob, *Iconografia d'anatomia*, 1841, vol. 2, pl. 16; **52 bl** Bourgery & Jacob, *Iconografia d'anatomia*, 1841, vol. 1, pl. 50; **52 br** Bourgery & Jacob, *Iconografia d'anatomia*, 1841, vol. 1, pl. 51; **53 all** Bourgery & Jacob, *Iconografia d'anatomia*, 1841, vol. 1, pl. 14; **54** Bernard & Huette, 1848, pl. 44 bis.; **55** Bernard & Huette, 1848, pl. 44; **56 all** Bourgery & Jacob, *Iconografia d'anatomia*, 1841, vol. 2, pl. 18; **57 tl, tr, cl** Bourgery & Jacob, *Iconografia d'anatomia*, 1841, vol. 2, pl. 16; **57 cr, bl, br** Bourgery & Jacob, *Iconografia d'anatomia*, 1841, vol. 2, pl. 17; **58** Bourgery & Jacob, *Iconografia d'anatomia*, 1841, vol. 1, pl. 64; **59** Bourgery & Jacob, *Iconografia d'anatomia*, 1841, vol. 1, pl. 65; **60** Joseph Pancoast, *A treatise on operative surgery comprising a description of the various processes of the art, including all the new operations; exhibiting the state of surgical science in its present advanced condition...*, Philadelphia, 1846, pl. 77; **61** Pancoast, 1846, pl. 4; **62 tl** Richard G. H. Butcher, *Reports in operative surgery*, Dublin, 1877, pl. xii; **62 tr** Butcher, 1877, pl. xiii; **62 bl** Butcher, 1877, pl. xiv; **62 br** Butcher, 1877, pl. xv; **63 tl** Butcher, 1877, pl. viii; **63 tr** Butcher, 1877, pl. ix; **63 bl** Butcher, 1877, pl. x; **63 br** Butcher, 1877, pl. xi; **64 fig. 1** Bernard & Huette, 1848, pl. 31; **fig. 2** Franz Anton, [A practitioner of Mesmerism using Animal Magnetism on a seated female patient], *c.* 1845, wood engraving; **fig. 3** John Snow, *On the inhalation of the vapour of ether in surgical operations*, London, 1847, p. 17; **65 fig. 4** *The London Medical Gazette or Journal of Practical Medicine*, London, 1847, vol. 6, p. 167; **fig. 5** Snow, 1847, p. 17; **fig. 6** F. R. Thomas, *Manual of the discovery, manufacture, and administration of nitrous oxide, or laughing gas*, Philadelphia, 1870, p. 72; **66 fig. 7** Charles Bell, *The anatomy and philosophy of expression as connected with the fine arts*, London, 1844, p. 157; **fig. 8** *A full discovery of the strange practices of Dr. Elliotson on the bodies of his female patients!...*, London, 1842, title page; **67 fig. 9** Frederic William Hewitt, *Anaesthetics and their administration: a manual for medical and dental practitioners and students*, London, 1893, p. 191; **fig. 10** Kvohne & Sesemann, *A catalogue of surgical instruments*, London, 1901, p. 335; **fig. 11** Bourgery & Jacob, *Traité complet de l'anatomie de l'homme*, 1839, vol. 6, pl. 85; **fig. 12** Hewitt, 1893, p. 191; **68 fig. 13** Unknown, [Sir James Y. Simpson & friends drink liquid chloroform in an experiment], *c.* 1840s, pen &

ink; **fig. 14** Dudley Wilmot Buxton, *Anæsthetics: their uses and administration*, London, 1900, p. 138; **fig. 15** Kvohne & Sesemann, *Illustrated catalogue of Surgical Instruments*, London, 1901, recto 331; **fig. 16** Kvohne & Sesemann, *A catalogue of surgical instruments*, London, 1901, p. 335; **69 fig. 17** Hewitt, 1922, p. 423; **70** Bourgery & Jacob, *Traité complet de l'anatomie de l'homme*, 1840, vol. 7, pl. B; **72–73** Bourgery & Jacob, *Iconografia d'anatomia*, 1841, vol. 2, pl. 2; **74** Bourgery & Jacob, *Traité complet de l'anatomie de l'homme*, 1840, vol. 7, pl. 4; **75** Bourgery & Jacob, *Traité complet de l'anatomie de l'homme*, 1840, vol. 7, pl. E; **76 l, c** G. J. Guthrie, *Lectures on the operative surgery of the eye...*, London, 1827, pl. 2; **76 r** G. J. Guthrie, 1827, pl. 3; **77 l** G. J. Guthrie, 1827, pl. 3; **77 c, r** G. J. Guthrie, 1827, pl. 7; **78** Bernard & Huette, 1848, pl. 39; **79** Bernard & Huette, 1848, pl. 40; **80 all** Bourgery & Jacob, *Iconografia d'anatomia*, 1841, vol. 2, pls. 5 & 6; **81 all** Bourgery & Jacob, *Iconografia d'anatomia*, 1841, vol. 2, pls. 7, 7 bis., 11; **82–83** Pancoast, 1846, pl. 49; **84 tl, tr** Bernard & Huette, 1848, pl. 41; **84 bl, br** Bernard & Huette, 1848, pl. 42; **85 tl** Bernard & Huette, 1848, pl. 42; **85 tr, bl** Bernard & Huette, 1848, pl. 41; **85 br** Bernard & Huette, 1848, pl. 42; **86** Bourgery & Jacob, *Iconografia d'anatomia*, 1841, vol. 2, pl. 10; **87** Bourgery & Jacob, *Iconografia d'anatomia*, 1841, vol. 2, pl. 9; **88 all** Bernard & Huette, 1848, pl. 37; **89 all** Bernard & Huette, 1848, pl. 36; **90 fig. 1** Robert Carswell, *Pathological anatomy: illustrations of the elementary forms of disease*, London 1838, pl. II; **fig. 2** C. Cook, [Florence Nightingale], stipple engraving; **fig. 3** Florence Nightingale, [Plan of the Barrack Hospital], *c.* 1855, in Western MS 5484, folio 13 recto; **91 fig. 4** A. W. Turnbull after R. A. Bickersteth, [Joseph Lister, 1ˢᵗ Baron Lister], etching; **fig. 5** Florence Nightingale, *Notes on hospitals*, London, 1863, pl. facing p. 112; **fig. 6** Unknown, [Portrait of Sir John Eric Erichsen], 1853, lithograph; **fig. 7** Henry Currey, *The Penny Illustrated Paper*, London, 9ᵗʰ May 1868, p. 300; **92 fig. 8** L. Orr, [Portrait of Louis Pasteur], etching; **fig. 9** Joseph Lister, "On the early stages of inflammation", *Philosophical transactions of the Royal Society of London*, 1858, vol. 148, part 2, p. 545; **fig. 10** W. Watson Cheyne, *Antiseptic Surgery: its principles, practice, history and results*, London, 1882, figs 55, 50, 49; **93 fig. 11** Joseph Lister, *The collected papers of Joseph, Baron Lister*, Oxford, 1909, vol. 1, pl. XI; **fig. 12** Lister family papers, [Advert for a Joseph Lister Lecture], 1857; **fig. 13** Watson Cheyne, 1882, fig. 38; **94 fig. 14** Unknown, [Bellevue Medical College, New York City], wood engraving; **fig. 15** Goodyear's India Rubber Manufacturing Co., [receipt], 1902, letterhead; **fig. 16** Unknown, [Robert Koch], 1891, lithograph; **fig. 17** Robert Koch, 'Zur untersuchung von pathogen organismen', *Collected Works*, vol. 1, pl. XVIII; **95 fig. 18** Watson Cheyne, 1882, fig. 23; **96** Bourgery & Jacob, *Traité complet de l'anatomie de l'homme*, 1836, vol. 4, pl. 26; **98–99** Bourgery & Jacob, *Iconografia d'anatomia*, 1841, vol. 2, pl. 19; **100 all** Bernard & Huette, 1848, pl. 43; **101 all** Bernard & Huette, 1848, pl. 43; **102 all** Bourgery & Jacob, *Traité complet de l'anatomie de l'homme*, 1840, vol. 7, pl. 12; **103 all** Bourgery & Jacob, *Traité complet de l'anatomie de l'homme*, 1840, vol. 7, pl. 15; **104** Bourgery & Jacob, *Iconografia d'anatomia*, 1841, vol. 2, pl. F; **105** Bourgery & Jacob, *Iconografia d'anatomia*, 1841, vol. 2, pl. G; **106 tl, tr** Bernard & Huette, 1848, pl. 47; **106 bl** Bernard & Huette, 1848, pl. 51; **106 br** Bernard & Huette, 1848, pl. 49; **107 tl** Bernard & Huette, 1848, pl. 47; **107 tr** Bernard & Huette, 1848, pl. 52; **107 bl** Bernard & Huette, 1848, pl. 47; **107 br** Bernard & Huette, 1848, pl. 49; **108–109** Bourgery & Jacob, *Traité complet de l'anatomie de l'homme*, 1840, vol. 7, pl. 24; **110** Pancoast, 1846, pl. 54; **111** Pancoast, 1846, pl. 55; **112** Christopher Heath, *A course of operative surgery with plates drawn from nature by M. Léveillé and coloured by hand under his direction*, London, 1877, pl. 10; **113** Heath, 1877, pl. 5; **114 tl** Bernard & Huette, 1848, pl. 46; **114 tc** Bernard & Huette, 1848, pl. 51 ter.; **110 tr** Bernard & Huette, 1848, pl. 47; **114 cl** Bernard & Huette, 1848, pl. 52; **114 c** Bernard & Huette, 1848, pl. 11; **114 cr, bl** Bernard & Huette, 1848, pl. 46; **114 bc** Bernard & Huette, 1848, pl. 51 ter.; **114 br** Bernard & Huette, 1848, pl. 48; **115 tl** Bernard & Huette, 1848, pl. 53; **115 tc** Bernard & Huette, 1848, pl. 38; **115 tr** Bernard & Huette, 1848, pl. 51 bis.; **115 cl** Bernard & Huette, 1848, pl. 52; **115 c** Bernard & Huette, 1848, pl. 53; **115 cr** Bernard & Huette, 1848, pl. 47; **115 bl** Bernard & Huette, 1848, pl. 53; **115 bc** Bernard & Huette, 1848, pl. 47; **115 br** Bernard & Huette, 1848, pl. 53; **116 fig. 1** J. Heuse, [Laparotomy operation at the Broca hospital, Paris], 1901, heliogravure; **fig. 2** Unknown, [Sir Frederick Treves], 1884, lithograph; **fig. 3** Watson Cheyne, 1882, fig. 23; **117 fig. 4** Karl Himly, *Die Krankheiten und Missbildungen des menschlichen Auges und deren Heilung*, Berlin, 1843, front cover; **fig. 5** F. C. Calvert & Co., [Magazine insert advertising F. C. Calvert's carbolic cleaning products], *c.* 1880s; **fig. 6** Robert Koch, "Investigations into the etiology of traumatic infective diseases", London, 1880; **118 fig. 7** Percy Frankland & Grace Coleridge Frankland, *Micro-organisms in water*, London, 1894, p. 2; **fig. 8** Watson Cheyne, 1882, fig. 25a; **fig. 9** *The Lancet*, 29ᵗʰ October 1892, p. 999; **119 fig. 10** *The Graphic*, 21ˢᵗ November 1885, p. 561; **fig. 11** Unknown, [The anatomy theatre at Padua], *c.* 1928, elevation; **fig. 12** Unknown, [The anatomy theatre at Padua], *c.* 1928, plan; **120 fig. 13** Arnold & Sons, *A catalogue of surgical instruments manufactured and sold by Arnold and Sons...*, London, 1873, p. 5; **fig. 14** Arnold & Sons, 1873, front cover; **fig. 15** *The Illustrated London News*, 1867, vol. 51, p. 245; **121 fig. 16** W. Koekkoek, *The Illustrated London News*, 1909, p. 557; **122** Bourgery & Jacob, *Traité complet de l'anatomie de l'homme*, 1839, vol. 6, pl. 76; **124–125** Bourgery & Jacob, *Iconografia d'anatomia*, 1841, vol. 1, pl. 27; **126 all** Bernard & Huette, 1848, pl. 12; **127 all** Bernard & Huette, 1848, pl. 7; **128 tl** Bernard & Huette, 1848, pl. 28; **128 tr** Bernard & Huette, 1848, pl. 19; **128 bl** bl Bernard & Huette, 1848, pl. 20; **128 br** Bernard & Huette, 1848, pl. 18; **129** Bernard & Huette, 1848, pl. 29; **130** Bourgery & Jacob, *Iconografia d'anatomia*, 1841, vol. 1, pl. 68; **131** Bourgery & Jacob, *Iconografia d'anatomia*, 1841, vol. 1, pl. 70; **132 all** Bourgery &

Jacob, *Traité complet de l'anatomie de l'homme*, 1839, vol. 6, pl. 69; **133 tl** Bourgery & Jacob, *Traité complet de l'anatomie de l'homme*, 1839, vol. 6, pl. 75; **133 tr, bl** Bourgery & Jacob, *Traité complet de l'anatomie de l'homme*, 1839, vol. 6, pl. 77; **133 br** Bourgery & Jacob, *Traité complet de l'anatomie de l'homme*, 1839, vol. 6, pl. 75; **134** Bernard & Huette, 1848, pl. 22; **135** Bernard & Huette, 1848, pl. 21; **136 tl** Pancoast, 1846, pl. 37; **136 tr** Pancoast, 1846, pl. 33; **136 bl** Pancoast, 1846, pl. 44; **136 br** Pancoast, 1846, pl. 28; **137 tl** Pancoast, 1846, pl. 29; **137 tr** Pancoast, 1846, pl. 35; **137 bl** Pancoast, 1846, pl. 39; **137 br** Pancoast, 1846, pl. 38; **138** Bourgery & Jacob, *Traité complet de l'anatomie de l'homme*, 1839, vol. 6, pl. 20; **139** Bourgery & Jacob, *Traité complet de l'anatomie de l'homme*, 1839, vol. 6, pl. 74; **140** Pancoast, 1846, pl. 7; **141** Pancoast, 1846, pl. 12; **142 fig. 1** Unknown, [Miss Elizabeth Garrett, M.D.], wood engraving; **fig. 2** F. Holl after Parthenope Nightingale, [Florence Nightingale], 1855, stipple engraving; **fig. 3** Unknown, [Sisters of Charity at the New Hospital at Pera, Turkey], *Illustrated London News*, wood engraving; **143 fig. 4** J. C. Buttre, [Elizabeth Fry], engraving; **fig. 5** Unknown, [Mrs Fry Visiting Newgate], reproduction of lithograph; **fig. 6** James Armytage, [Miss Nightingale & the nurses in the East], line engraving; **fig. 7** Alexis Soyer, *Soyer's culinary campaign...*, London, 1857; **144 fig. 8** Florence Nightingale, *A contribution to the sanitary history of the British army during the late war with Russia*, London, 1859; **fig. 9** Royal Commission Appointed to Enquire into the Sanitary Condition of the Army, *Mortality of the British army at home and abroad...*, London, 1858, courtesy of The RAMC Muniment Collection in the care of the Wellcome Library; **fig. 10** Florence Nightingale, *A contribution to the sanitary history of the British army during the late war with Russia*, London, 1859; **fig. 11** Sarah A. Tooley, *The life and times of Florence Nightingale*, London, 1904, p. 237; **145 fig. 12** Unknown, [Florence Nightingale], 1854, lithograph; **fig. 13** Unknown, [An Army matron from the General Hospital, Dar-es-salaam], lithograph; **fig. 14** G. Villanova, [Operation for vaginal hysterectomy], heliogravure; **146 fig. 15** Honnor Morten, *How to become a nurse and how to succeed*, London, 1892; **fig. 16** after William Henman & Thomas Cooper, [Royal Victoria Hospital, Belfast: a visit by the King & Queen...], 1903, pen & ink; **fig. 17** George Du Maurier, cartoon in Punch, London; **147 fig. 18** Queen's Nursing Institute, [cover of booklet on the Liverpool Queen Victoria District Nursing Association]; **148** Bourgery & Jacob, *Traité complet de l'anatomie de l'homme*, 1836, vol. 4, pl. 8; **150–151** Bourgery & Jacob, *Iconografia d'anatomia*, 1841, vol. 1, pl. 17; **152** Bernard & Huette, 1848, pl. 9; **153** Bernard & Huette, 1848, pl. 10; **154** Maclise, 1856, pl. 14; **155** Bernard & Huette, 1848, pl. 1; **156** Bernard & Huette, 1848, pl. 54; **157** Heath, 1877, pl. 4; **158** Bourgery & Jacob, *Iconografia d'anatomia*, 1841, vol. 2, pl. 27; **159** Bourgery & Jacob, *Iconografia d'anatomia*, 1841, vol. 2, pl. 28; **160 fig. 1** Unknown, [The Morning After the Battle of Inkerman], 1854, wood engraving; **fig. 2** Henry Walker, "The Rifle Fever", song sheet; **161 fig. 3** *Illustrated London News*, 1860, vol. 36, p. 53; **fig. 4** William Turnbull, *The naval surgeon; comprising the entire duties of professional men at sea...*, London, 1806, pl. 1: **fig. 5** Turnbull, 1806, pl. 2; **162 fig. 6** J. H. Porter, *The surgeon's pocket-book*, London, 1875, fig. 45; **fig. 7** Turnbull, 1806, pl. 6; **fig. 8** Irving Montagu, *The Illustrated London News*, 10ᵗʰ November 1877, p. 446; **163 fig. 9** Charles William Sheeres, *The Illustrated London News*, 17ᵗʰ March 1855, p. 244; **fig. 10** LEA. W. [Crimean War, England: receiving lint to be sent to Scutari], wood engraving; **fig. 11** Francois Le Villain, [A soldier having an arm amputated], lithograph; **164 fig. 12** William MacCormac, *Antiseptic surgery...*, London, 1880, p. 274; **fig. 13** T. Longmore, *A treatise on the transport of sick and wounded troups*, London, 1869, fig. XLVII; **fig. 14** *The Illustrated London News*, 30ᵗʰ December 1854, p. 693; **fig. 15** Allan Powell, *The Metropolitan Asylums Board and its Work 1867-1930*, London, 1930, facing p. 78; **165 fig. 16** Unknown, [Crimean War: ambulance men removing the wounded from the Battle of Sebastopol] c. 1854, wood engraving; **166** Bourgery & Jacob, *Traité complet de l'anatomie de l'homme*, 1839, vol. 6, pl. 26; **168–169** Bourgery & Jacob, *Iconografia d'anatomia*, 1841, vol. 2, pl. 16; **170 t** Bernard & Huette, 1848, pl. 17; **170 b** Bernard & Huette, 1848, pl. 62 ter.; **171 tl, tr** Bernard & Huette, 1848, pl. 54 bis.; **171 bl, br** Bernard & Huette, 1848, pl. 62 bis.; **172–173** Bourgery & Jacob, *Traité complet de l'anatomie de l'homme*, 1840, vol. 7, pl. 40; **174** Bourgery & Jacob, *Iconografia d'anatomia*, 1841, vol. 2, pl. 32; **175** Bourgery & Jacob, *Iconografia d'anatomia*, 1841, vol. 2, pl. 33; **176** Bernard & Huette, 1848, pl. 63; **177** Bernard & Huette, 1848, pl. 63 bis.; **178–179** Bourgery & Jacob, *Iconografia d'anatomia*, 1841, vol. 2, pl. 29; **180** Bourgery & Jacob, *Traité complet de l'anatomie de l'homme*, 1840, vol. 7, pl. 77; **181** Bourgery & Jacob, *Traité complet de l'anatomie de l'homme*, 1840, vol. 7, pl. 77; **182 fig. 1** Richard Quain & Joseph Maclise, *The anatomy of the arteries of the human body: with its applications to pathology and operative surgery*, London, 1844, vol. 2, pl. 1; **fig. 2** Unknown, [Medical College & Charity Hospital, New York City], coloured wood engraving; **fig. 3** E. Grünewald after B. Kundeshagen, [A view of the Anatomy theatre & University buildings, Bonn, Germany], line engraving; **183 fig. 4** [Card admitting Robert Lee to medical course], 1822; **fig. 5** D. D. Dobree, [Notes on John Abernethy's lectures on anatomy, physiology, etc.], c. 1814; **fig. 6** William Hunter, *Historical Account of Charing Cross Hospital and Medical School*, London, 1914, pl. XXXVII; **184 fig. 7** Jacques-Pierre Maygrier, *Nouvelles démonstrations d'accouchemens*, Paris, 1822 pl. LXIV; **fig. 8** Maygrier, 1822 pl. LXXVI; **fig. 9** Achille Louis Foville, *Traité complet de l'anatomie, de la physiologie, et de la pathologie du système nerveux cérébro-spinal...*, Paris, 1844, pl. 9; **185, fig. 10** Swift & Son, *Swift & Son's new patent microscope*, London, c. 1890; **fig. 11** Swift & Son, c. 1890; **fig. 12** Etienne Jules Marey, *La methode graphique dans les sciences experimentales*, Paris, 1878, p. 614; **186 fig. 13** Unknown, *Traite de Microscope*, Paris, 1871, fig. 65; **fig. 14** Bourgery & Jacob, *Traité complet de l'anatomie* *de l'homme*, 1831-1854 vol. 3, pl. 88; **fig. 15** Bourgery & Jacob, *Traité complet de l'anatomie de l'homme*, 1831-1854, vol. 3, pl. 88 bis.; **187 fig. 16**; George Gladwin after B. Dixie, [Interior of the theatre of the London Institution], etching; **188** Bourgery & Jacob, *Traité complet de l'anatomie de l'homme*, 1840, vol. 7, pl. 72; **190-191** Bourgery & Jacob, *Iconografia d'anatomia*, 1841, vol. 2, pl. 54; **192 t** Bernard & Huette, 1848, pl. 67; **192 b** Bernard & Huette, 1848, pl. 68; **193 all** Bernard & Huette, 1848, pl. 57; **194** Bernard & Huette, 1848, pl. 64; **195** Bernard & Huette, 1848, pl. 69; **196** Bourgery & Jacob, *Iconografia d'anatomia*, 1841, vol. 2, pl. 57 bis.; **197** Bourgery & Jacob, *Iconografia d'anatomia*, 1841, vol. 2, pl. 60; **198** Bernard & Huette, 1848, pl. 65; **199** Bernard & Huette, 1848, pl. 66; **200-201** Bourgery & Jacob, *Iconografia d'anatomia*, 1841, vol. 2, pl. 26; **202** Henry Savage, *The surgery, surgical pathology and surgical anatomy of the female pelvic organs...*, London, 1882, pl. 4; **203** Savage, 1882, pl. 7; **204** Bernard & Huette, 1848, pl. 76; **205 all** Bernard & Huette, 1848, pl. 73; **206 tl** Savage, 1882, pl. 13; **206 tr** Savage, 1882, pl. 10; **206 bl** Savage, 1882, pl. 6; **206 br** Savage, 1882, pl. 10; **207 tl** Savage, 1882, pl. 13; **207 tr, bl** Savage, 1882, pl. 12; **207 br** Savage, 1882, pl. 13; **208** Bernard & Huette, 1848, pl. 75; **209** Savage, 1882, pl. 14; **210 fig. 1** after Joshua Reynolds, [John Hunter], c. 1900, oil painting; **fig. 2** Charles Bell, *Illustrations of the Great Operations of Surgery*, London, 1820-1821, pl. 2; **fig. 3** H. M. Paget after W. T. Maud, *Illustrated London News*; **211 fig. 4** Unknown, [Theodor Kocher], photogravure; **fig. 5** after Franz Lenbach, [Theodor Billroth], 1884, gravure; **fig. 6** Thomas Godart [Dissected right knee joint showing tubercular synovitis], 1886, watercolour drawing; **212 fig. 7** Grove Son & Boulton, [John Hunter's residence], 1832, photoprint; **213 fig. 8** Jesse Foot, *The Life of John Hunter*, London, 1822, vol. 2, p. 222; **fig. 9** James Paget, "On a form of chronic inflammation of bones (Osteitis deformans)", *Medic-chirurgical transactions*, 1877, figs. 1-3; **fig. 10** [First aid kit belonging to King Edward VII], 1904; **214 fig. 11** Hugh Owen Thomas, *Diseases of the hip, knee, and ankle, joints, with their deformities, treated by a new and efficient method*, Liverpool, 1876, figs. 4 & 6; **fig. 12** Thomas, 1876; **215 fig. 13** Augustus Fox after T. H. Shepherd, [Hunterian Museum, Glasgow], 1830, line engraving; **216** Bourgery & Jacob, *Traité complet de l'anatomie de l'homme*, 1839, vol. 6, pl. 21; **218-219** Bourgery & Jacob, *Iconografia d'anatomia*, 1841, vol. 1, pl. 55; **220** Bourgery & Jacob, *Traité complet de l'anatomie de l'homme*, 1839, vol. 6, pl. 83; **221** Bourgery & Jacob, *Traité complet de l'anatomie de l'homme*, 1839, vol. 6, pl. 83 bis.; **222 tl** Bernard & Huette, 1848, pl. 30; **222 tr, bl** Bernard & Huette, 1848, pl. 27; **222 br** Bernard & Huette, 1848, pl. 30; **223 tl** Bernard & Huette, 1848, pl. 31; **223 tr** Bernard & Huette, 1848, pl. 33; **223 bl** Bernard & Huette, 1848, pl. 27; **223 br** Bernard & Huette, 1848, pl. 33; **224 tl** Bourgery & Jacob, *Traité complet de l'anatomie de l'homme*, 1839, vol. 6, pl. 85; **224 tr, bl** Bourgery & Jacob, *Traité complet de l'anatomie de l'homme*, 1839, vol. 6, pl. 88; **224 br** Bourgery & Jacob, *Traité complet de l'anatomie de l'homme*, 1839, vol. 6, pl. 89; **225 tl, tr** Bourgery & Jacob, *Traité complet de l'anatomie de l'homme*, 1839, vol. 6, pl. 90; **225 bl** Bourgery & Jacob, *Traité complet de l'anatomie de l'homme*, 1839, vol. 6, pl. 89; **225 br** Bourgery & Jacob, *Traité complet de l'anatomie de l'homme*, 1839, vol. 6, pl. 85; **226** Heath, 1877, pl. 17; **227** Heath, 1877, pl. 18; **228 tl** Bernard & Huette, 1848, pl. 15; **228 tc** Bernard & Huette, 1848, pl. 25; **228 tr** Bernard & Huette, 1848, pl. 26; **228 cl, c** Bernard & Huette, 1848, pl. 25; **228 cr** Bernard & Huette, 1848, pl. 15; **228 bl** Bernard & Huette, 1848, pl. 28; **228 bc, br** Bernard & Huette, 1848, pl. 25; **229 tl** Bernard & Huette, 1848, pl. 15; **229 tc** Bernard & Huette, 1848, pl. 12; **229 tr** Bernard & Huette, 1848, pl. 4; **229 cl** Bernard & Huette, 1848, pl. 28; **229 c** Bernard & Huette, 1848, pl. 15; **229 bl** Bernard & Huette, 1848, pl. 4; **229 bc** Bernard & Huette, 1848, pl. 26; **230 all** Joseph K. Barnes, *The medical and surgical history of the war of the rebellion, (1861-65)*, Washington, 1888, pl. LXXXV; **231** George Alexander Otis, *A report on amputations at the hip-joint in military surgery*, Washington, 1867, "Blackman's successful amputation at the hip-joint"; **232 all** Barnes, 1888, pl. LXXIIII; **233 t** Otis, 1867, "Shippen's successful primary amputation at the hip joint"; **233 c** Otis, 1867, "Packard's successful re-amputation at the hip joint"; **233 b** Barnes, 1888, pl. IX; **234** Otis, 1867, "Morton's successful re-amputation at the hip joint"; **235** Otis, 1867, "Mott's successful re-amputation at the hip joint"; **236** Bourgery & Jacob, *Iconografia d'anatomia*, 1841, vol. 1, pl. 80; **237** Bourgery & Jacob, *Iconografia d'anatomia*, 1841, vol. 1, pl. 81; **238** N. H. Jacob, loose leaf, plate to Bourgery & Jacob, *Traité complet de l'anatomie de l'homme*, 1831-1854, vol. 7, pl. J; **239 all** Pancoast, 1846, pl. 79; **240 fig. 1** P. Simonau after Charles Le Brun, [a face turned away, suffering acute pain], 1822, lithograph; **fig. 2** Alexander Morrison and Byrom Bramwell, [A woman diagnosed as suffering from melancholia with fear], 1892, lithograph; **241 fig. 3** Pancoast, 1846, pl. 37; **fig. 4** Pancoast, 1846, pl. 37; **fig. 5** Electropathic & Zander Institute, [advertisement for therapeutic belts], c. 1890s, magazine insert or leaflet; **242 fig. 6** Paul Marie Louis Pierre Richer, *Etudes cliniques sur l'hystero-epilepsie ou grande hysterie*, Paris, 1881, pl. III; **fig. 7** Richer, 1881, pl. IV; **243 fig. 8** Samuel Auguste Andre David Tissot, *L'onanisme; ou dissertation physique sur les maladies produites par la masturbation*, Paris, 1836, frontispiece & plate preceding page 1; **fig. 9** G. Jalade-Lafond, *Considerations sur les Herenies Abdominales, sur les Bandages Herniaries Renixigrades et sur de Nouveaux Moyens de S'Opposer A l'Onanisme*, Paris, 1822, vol. 1, pl. 12; **fig. 10** Jalade-Lafond, 1822, vol. 1, pl. 15; **244 fig. 11** Thomas Spencer Wells, *Diseases of the ovaries: their diagnosis and treatment*, London, 1865, p. 340; **fig. 12** *Catalogue and Report of Obstetrical and Other instruments exhibited at the Conversazione of the Obstetrical Society of London*, London, 1867, pp. 139-140; **fig. 13** Watson Cheyne, 1882, fig. 36; **245 fig. 14** Hewitt, 1893, fig. 43; **256** Bourgery & Jacob, *Traité complet de l'anatomie de l'homme*, 839, vol. 6, pl. 28.

INDEX

Illustrations are in **bold**.

abdomen
    dissection **11**, **166**,
        170-1
    peritoneal tap **178-9**
Académie Royale de
    Chirurgie, foundation
    39
accoucheurs 39-40
ambulances 164
amputations
    arm **122**, **129**, **133-7**,
        139, 163-4, **241**
    fingers **128**, **130-2**,
        136-7
    foot 162, **227-9**, **236-7**
    hand **128**
    leg **13**, 16, **64**, **67**,
        220-7, **229-35**
    penis **198**
    toes **128**, **227**, **229**
anaesthesia 16, 22-3, **45**,
    64-8, **69**, 163
Anathomia Mundini
    (Mondino) **28**
*Anatomia Corporis
    Humani* (Mondino)
    29-30
anatomo-localism 41,
    43-4, 183-4
anatomy schools 39
Anglo-Saxon surgery 22
antisepsis 90-4, **95**,
    116-17, 144-5, 164
Apothecaries Act 1815 183
appendectomy 213-14
arm surgery **122**, **126-7**,
    129, **133-7**, **139**, **152**,
    163-4, **241**
Ars Computistica
    (Heymandus) **31**
arteries
    compression 46, **138**,
        141, **216**
    incisions **61**
    ligatures 4-5, **113**,
        114, **126-7**, **136**,
        140, **153**, 229
Arzneibuch **26-7**
asepsis 116-20, **121**
Avicenna 21

Baghdad 21
Baker Brown, Isaac 243
Bamberg surgery 24
Bartisch, George **24-5**
Barton, Clara 144
Battey, Robert 243
Beddoes, Thomas 65

Behzad, Husayn **22**
Bell, Charles **66**
Bichat, Xavier 43, 44
Billroth, Theodor 184, 211
Binns, Joseph 32
Blackwell, Elizabeth 242
bladder
    lithotomy 38, 41
    lithotripsy **168-9**,
        172-3, **196-7**
    surgical puncture **192**
bloodletting 21, 22, **30**, 44
Boy Scouts (Baden-
    Powell) 164
Braid, James 66-7
brain **50-1**, **184**
Branca family 27
breast pump **124**
breast surgery **156-8**,
    243-4
Brown, John 65

Cabanis, Pierre 43
caesarean section **180-1**,
    184
Caius, John 30
Callender, George
    William 93
carbolic acid 92, 93-4,
    117-18
Carrel, Alexis 211
cataracts 41, **76**, **77**, **84-7**
catheters **190-1**, **192**, **197**
Celsus, Cornelius 19, **21**
Chamberlen family 27
Chaucer 23, 25
Chauliac, Guy de 26
Cheselden, William
    40, 41
chest, dissection **148**,
    154-5
Chirurgia Magna
    (Chauliac) 26
*Chirurgische
    Operationslehre* (Kocher)
    211
chloroform 68, 163
Classical tradition 19-21,
    26, 30
cleft lip/palate correction
    48-9, **54-6**, **62**, **106**,
    107, **111**
Clowes, William 33, 35
club foot **238-9**
cocaine 68
collaboration 185-6
Colot family 27
Company of Barber-
    Surgeons 23, 31
Company of Surgeons 39
conservatism 19, 21, 27,
    31, 213, 214
consumption 65-6
control ideology 118-19
Cooper, Astley 44
cupping instruments
    124-5
Cushing, Harvey 211

Dalton, John 67
Davy, Humphry 65
*De Humani Corporis
    Fabrica* (Vesalius) 31-2
De Medicina (Celsus)
    19, **21**
*De Sedibus et Causis
    Morborum* (Morgagni)
    43
Deaver, John 214
Dennis, Frederick 210-11
Descartes, René 41
Dieffenbach, Johann
    Friedrich 240-1
Dionis, Pierre 38
dislocations **37**
dissections
    18th century **40**
    abdomen **11**, **166**,
        170-1
    brain **184**
    chest **148**, **154-5**
    female genitals **205**,
        206, **207**
    female reproductive
        system **202-3**
    leg **228**
    male genitals **193**
    medieval **17**, **28**, 29-31
    trunk **11**
Dix, Dorothea 144
dwale 22-3

ear surgery **100-2**
Eichhorn, Gerhard 32-3
elbow, dislocation **37**
elitism 18, 185
Elliotson, John 66
empyema drainage **156**,
    159
erysipelas 90
ether 64, 66, 67
eyes
    artificial pupil **77**, **81**
    cataracts 41, **76**, **77**,
        84-7
    eyelids **76**, **77**, **80-1**,
        88-9
    glaucoma **77**
    immobilisation **70**
    lacrimal system
        74, **78**
    medieval surgery
        24-5, **26-7**
    muscles **79**
    sclera **79**
    strabismus **75**, **82-3**

Fabricius, Hieronymus
    16, 18
facial injury repair **57**
Fagon, Guy-Crescent 38
Fasciculus Medicinae
    (Ketham) **16**, **17**
Félix, C. F. 38
Fellowship of Surgeons,
    establishment 23
female genitals *see*

also genital surgery,
    dissections **205**, **206**,
    207
female reproductive
    system, dissections
    202-3
fingers, amputations **128**,
    130-2, **136-7**
Fliedner, Theodor 143
foot surgery 162, **216**, **227**,
    228-9, **236-9**
Fry, Elizabeth 143

Gale, Thomas 26
Galen, Claudius 19, 26, 31
gangrene 90, 92
Garrett Anderson,
    Elizabeth 142
General Nursing Council
    145
genital surgery *see also*
    bladder
    instruments **190-1**,
        200-1
    penis **194-5**, **198**
    perineum **206**, **207**
    testis **199**
    uterus **188**, **208**
    vagina **209**
germ theory 92, **93**, 94,
    117, 118
glaucoma **77**
goitre removal **96**, **114**,
    184
gonorrhoea 33
Graefer, Albrecht 184
Gray, H. M. W. 164
Gregory, John 42
Gretter, Lystra E. 144
*Guide to the Aseptic
    Treatment of Wounds*
    (Schimmelbusch) 118
guilds 23-4

haemorrhoids **177**
Hall, Sir John 163
Halle, John 32
Haller, Albrecht von 43
Halsted, William 93, 243
hand, prosthetic **36**
hand surgery **126-8**,
    130-2, **136-7**
hare-lip *see* cleft lip/palate
    correction
Harte, Richard A. 214
Harvey, William 18, 32
head surgery **46-63**
Heymandus de Veteri
    Busco **31**
Hickman, Henry Hill 66
Hippocratic Corpus 19
hospitals
    18th century 40
    antisepsis 90
    medieval
        development 28
    military 161
    mortality rates 90-1

Paris 42-3
pavilion-hospitals 90-1
specialization 184-5
House of Wisdom, Baghdad 21
humours 19
Hunter, John 41, **210**, 211-13, **215**
Hunter, William 39

incisions **6-7**, **61**, 120, **150-1**
Instrumenta Chyrurgiae et Icones Anathomicae (Paré) **36-7**
instruments
    bone operations **218-19**
    cauterizaton **150-1**
    cleft lip/palate correction **48-9**
    cupping **124-5**
    ear surgery **100**, **101**
    eye surgery **72-3**
    female reproductive system **200-1**, **204**
    incisions **150-1**
    male genito-urinary system **190-1**
    military surgery **33**, **36**, **162**
    mouth surgery **106-7**
    nasal surgery **103**
    specialization 119-20, 185
    suturing needles **2**
    throat surgery **98-9**, **104-5**, **108-9**
    wound dressing **150-1**
intestinal surgery **170**, **171**, **174-5**
Islamic Golden Age 21

jaw resection **58-9**
Jones, Robert 214
journals, development of 184, 185

Ketham, Johannes de 16, **17**
Kheirourgos 19
kidney, lithotripsy **168-9**, **172-3**
Koch, Robert 94, 117-18
Kocher, Emil Theodor 118, 184, 211
Koller, Carl 68
Kymer, Gilbert 24

laboratory development 185-6
Lane, William Arbuthnot 242
Larrey, Dominique-Jean 243

Lawson Tait, Robert 94
Le Brun, Charles **240**
Leechbook of Bald 22
leg
    amputation **13**, 16, **220-7**, **229-35**
    arterial compression **216**
    dissections **228**
    prosthetic **37**
    Thomas splint 214
Lister, Joseph 18, 90, 91-2, 94, 117-18, 211, 213
Liston, Robert 44-5, 67
lithotomy 38, 41
lithotripsy **168-9**, **172-3**, **196-7**

Macleod, George 160
male genitals *see also* genital surgery, dissections **193**
Mareschal, Georges 38
mastectomy **156-8**, 243-4
matrons 144, 145
McDowell, Ephraim 243
medieval surgery 16, 18, **20**
mesmerism 64, 66-7
Methodus Medendi (Galen) 19
miasma 91
microscopes 185
midwifery 39-40
military surgery 33-5, 40, 120, 160-4, **165**, **230-1**, **233**, **235**
monasteries 22, 28
Mondino de Luzzi **28**, 29-30
Morgagni, Giovanni Battista 43, 44
mortality rates 16, 90-1, **144**
Morton, William 64, 67
mouth surgery **106-11**, **114**, **115**
Moynihan, Berkeley 118
muscles, tenotomy **8-9**

naval surgery *see* military surgery
Nightingale, Florence 90, 91, 142, 143-4
nitrous oxide 65-6, 67
Nobel Prize 211
noses
    artificial **35**
    surgery **53**, **103**, **114**
Notes on Nursing (Nightingale) 144
nursing 142-6, **147**

operating theatres
    asepsis 116-20, **121**
    nurses 144-5
Ophthalmodouleia (Bartisch) **24-5**

oral surgery *see* mouth surgery
Osler, Sir William 213
ovaries **202-3**

Paget, James 212, **213**
pain 65, 66, 163, 241-2, 244
Paré, Ambroise **34**, 35, **36-7**, 41
Paris medicine 42-4, 182
Pasteur, Louis 92, 117
pathology 185-6
patient's perspective 240-4
penis **194-5**
peritoneal tap **178-9**
Pneumatic Institute, Bristol 65
Priestley, Joseph 65
prosthetics
    hands **36**
    leg **37**
    nose **35**

rectum **176-7**
Red Cross 164
Rhazes 21, **22**
rhinoplasty **53**
Robinson, James 67
Royal College of Physicians **39**
Royal College of Surgeons 39, 212
Royal Nursing Association 145

Salvation Army 164
Schimmelbusch, Curt 118
shoulder **37**, **153**, **157**
Simpson, James Young 68, 90-1
Sims, James Marion 243
sinuses perforation **52**
skin **2**, **186**
skull **52**
Smellie, William 39
Snow, John 67, 68
specialization 183-5
sphygmomanometer 185
Spurzheim, Johann Gaspar 64
St John Ambulance Brigade 164
stammering 240-1
steam sterilization 118
Studies on the Aetiology of Wound Infection (Koch) 117
surgeon-apothecaries 41, 43, 120
surgeons
    16th-17th centuries 30-5
    18th century 38-42
    20th century beginnings 210-14

classical 19
early 19th century 44-5
medieval 16, 18, 21, 23-8
sutures, skin **2**
Syntagma Anatomicum (Vesling) **14**
syphilis 33

Tagliacozzi, Gaspare 33
teaching surgery **121**, 182-6, **187**
tendons **8-9**
Tenon, Jacques-René 91
tenotomy **8-9**
testis **199**
The Anatomy and Philosophy of Expression (Bell) **66**
Thomas, Hugh Owen 214
Thompson, John 161
throat surgery **96**, **104-6**, **108-9**, **111-15**
toes, amputations **128**, **227**, **229**
tongue **106-7**, **110**, **114**, **115**, 240-1
tonsils **114**
Topham, William 64
Todd Crawford, Jane 243
Townend, Joseph 240
trachea **104-5**, **106**, **108-9**, **111**, **112**, **115**
transplants 211
Treves, Frederick 116, 213
tumour removal **63**, **101-2**, **115**, **198**, 243

universities, European establishment 23-5
uterus **188**, **202-3**, **204**, **208**

vagina **202-3**, **209**
venereal diseases 33, 184
Vesalius, Andreas 31-2
Vesling, Johann **14**

Ward, W. Squire 64
'Wellcome Apocalypse' **30**
Wells, T. S. 93
Wiseman, Richard 32, 35
women
    as nurses 142-6
    as patients 242-4 *see also* genital surgery
Woodall, John 35
wound management
    antisepsis 92-4
    classical theory 21, 26
    incision improvements 120
    Paré, Ambroise 35, **36**
'Wound Men' **20**, 31
Wrench, Edward 164

'Zodiac Men' **29**, 31

ABOUT THE AUTHOR

Richard Barnett has taught the cultural history of science and medicine at the universities of London and Cambridge, and in 2011 received one of the first Wellcome Trust Engagement Fellowships. His most recent book, *The Sick Rose: Disease and the Art of Medical Illustration*, was described by Will Self as 'superbly erudite and lucid'. Find him online at richardbarnettwriter.com.

Subcutaneous cupping devices for the arm and leg, intended to draw blood to the skin so that it could be released by scarification.

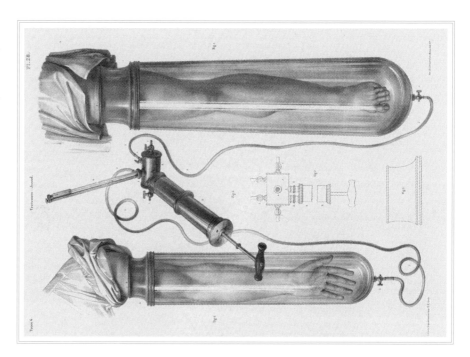

ACKNOWLEDGMENTS

For their professional contributions, thanks to Tristan de Lancey, Jane Laing, Charlie Mounter, Jon Crabb & Rose Blackett-Ord at Thames & Hudson; Peter Robinson & Federica Leonardis at Rogers, Coleridge & White; Simon Chaplin, Phoebe Harkins, & Ross MacFarlane at the Wellcome Library; Catherine Draycott, Crestina Forcina & Kathleen Arundell at Wellcome Images; & Ken Arnold & Kirty Topiwala at Wellcome Collection. For their friendship & patience, thanks to Paul Craddock, Patricia Hammond, Roger Kneebone, Michael Neve, & Kelley Swain.

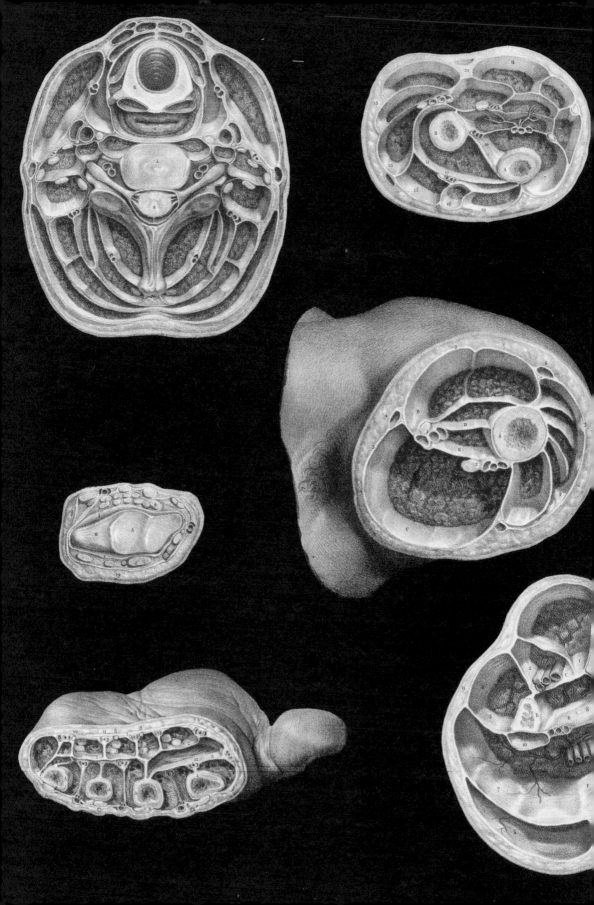

60 0098842 4   TELEPEN

WITHDRAWN

Students and External Readers	Staff & Research Students
DATE DUE FOR RETURN	**DATE OF ISSUE**

26. JUN 85 0 5 0

-9 DEC 85 0 0 0

29. JUN 94

- 3 FEB 1987

ONE WEEK ONLY

FOUR WEEKS ONLY

3 1 JAN 1989

19 XXXXX 90   - 6 FEB 1997

18. MAR 91

09. FEB 95

28. 06 95

28. 06 95

28. 06 95

N.B. All books must be returned for the Annual Inspection in June

Any book which you borrow remains your responsibility until the loan slip is cancelled